W9-BJF-690

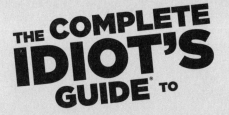
THE COMPLETE IDIOT'S GUIDE TO

Gluten-Free Vegan Cooking

by Julieanna Hever, M.S., R.D., C.P.T., and Beverly Lynn Bennett

15 September 17

Happy Healthy Cooking, David!

Julieanna Hever

A
ALPHA
A member of Penguin Group (USA) Inc.

This book is dedicated to all the gluten-free vegans who have struggled to find something tasty to eat—this one's for you!

ALPHA BOOKS

Published by the Penguin Group

Penguin Group (USA) Inc., 375 Hudson Street, New York, New York 10014, USA

Penguin Group (Canada), 90 Eglinton Avenue East, Suite 700, Toronto, Ontario M4P 2Y3, Canada (a division of Pearson Penguin Canada Inc.)

Penguin Books Ltd., 80 Strand, London WC2R 0RL, England

Penguin Ireland, 25 St. Stephen's Green, Dublin 2, Ireland (a division of Penguin Books Ltd.)

Penguin Group (Australia), 250 Camberwell Road, Camberwell, Victoria 3124, Australia (a division of Pearson Australia Group Pty. Ltd.)

Penguin Books India Pvt. Ltd., 11 Community Centre, Panchsheel Park, New Delhi—110 017, India

Penguin Group (NZ), 67 Apollo Drive, Rosedale, North Shore, Auckland 1311, New Zealand (a division of Pearson New Zealand Ltd.)

Penguin Books (South Africa) (Pty.) Ltd., 24 Sturdee Avenue, Rosebank, Johannesburg 2196, South Africa

Penguin Books Ltd., Registered Offices: 80 Strand, London WC2R 0RL, England

Publisher: *Marie Butler-Knight*
Associate Publisher: *Mike Sanders*
Executive Managing Editor: *Billy Fields*
Senior Acquisitions Editor: *Tom Stevens*
Senior Development Editor: *Christy Wagner*
Senior Production Editor: *Kayla Dugger*

Copy Editor: *Monica Stone*
Cover Designer: *Rebecca Batchelor*
Book Designers: *William Thomas, Rebecca Batchelor*
Indexer: *Celia McCoy*
Layout: *Ayanna Lacey*
Senior Proofreader: *Laura Caddell*

Contents

Appendixes

Introduction

What an exciting time to be gluten free and vegan! The tides have shifted as more and more people grow increasingly aware of the impact food has on their bodies and on the world around them. Information and support are abundant, as well as carefully manufactured food products geared toward your pleasure, ethics, and safety. No longer do you have to fend for yourself in order to prevent an accidental consumption of gluten or animal product. Labeling laws have simplified your purchasing concerns, and restaurants are alerted to the seriousness of food allergies.

Chance and luck are not dictating why this revolution is occurring. Instead, there has been a large increase in gluten and other food intolerances in recent years. After decades of indulging in a diet based on highly processed, refined, junk, and fast foods, our bodies are catching up and rebelling. Although the majority of intolerances are not due to celiac sprue or allergy, a huge chunk of the general population now suffers with discomforting and painful symptoms. Thus, between all intolerant origins (including allergy and celiac sprue), a vast bulk of people need to focus more carefully on the foods they consume at each meal.

Fortunately, gluten free and vegan is not a taste bud death sentence. On the contrary, a flavorful world exists, reaching far beyond what you may have imagined. Together, with our nutritional and culinary expertise, we are thrilled to offer you more than 200 recipes that will tantalize your palate and provide you with creative and delicious options you can easily create at home. From appetizers to desserts and breakfast to dinner, we take you on a culinary excursion through unique dishes you may never have seen before, to classics you probably thought you needed to part with forever. Get ready to open your eyes and lips for a gluten-free vegan extravaganza!

How This Book Is Organized

This book is divided into six parts, devoted to showing you how easy—and delicious!—a gluten-free vegan diet can be:

Part 1, Living Gluten Free and Vegan, offers a comprehensive course in gluten-free and vegan basics, explaining the health advantages of omitting gluten and animal products from your diet and providing you with guidelines to help you do so. We show you how to easily substitute plant-based and gluten-free ingredients to make any recipe you like, and help you equip your kitchen so you can be ready to create whenever the mood strikes.

Part 2, Off to a Good Start, lays the foundation for starting off your day right by providing you with recipes for quick and easy breakfast, as well as a few classic brunch selections. You also learn how to make several gluten-free and vegan sweet and savory baked goods, breads, buns, and pie and pizza crusts. We end this part with a DIY guide to making your own vegan cheeses.

Part 3, Snacks, Sauces, and Spreads, features recipes for healthy snacking options, fantastic appetizers, and other finger foods. We then move on to savory spreads, hummus, pâtés, and everyone's favorite guacamole and salsa, all of which are perfect for pairing with crunchy dippers. We finish up with an array of sauces, and we've got you covered whether you're in need of some gravy; pesto; or a sweet, spicy, or creamy sauce.

In **Part 4, Ready for Lunch?,** we show you how to grow your own sprouts, mix up some crunchy veggie-packed slaws, make two types of potato salads, and pull together delicious and nutritious tossed and leafy green salads. We also teach you how to make, bake, and steam your own meatless meats and provide ideas for utilizing them in filling and hearty sandwiches. And forget about opening up a can because our soup, stew, chili, and chowder recipes are far superior in terms of flavor and ingredients used than those tinned varieties.

Part 5, Exceptional Entrées and Side Dishes, contains main and side dish recipes you'll love to serve your family and friends. Whatever your mood or appetite, we've got something in these chapters that's sure to appeal to you, whether you want pizza, pasta, Mexican, Asian, or Indian—or enough-for-an-army casserole. And to nicely round out your dinner plate, we've also included an endless array of tasty grain-, bean-, and veggie-based side dishes.

Part 6, Divine Desserts, shows you how to make and bake some delectable and divine desserts. You learn how to make scrumptious cookies, brownies, and bars, plus pies and tarts, puddings, tasty toppings, assorted cakes and cupcakes, and cheesecake. Whatever your sweet tooth is craving, you'll surely find something to your liking in this part. Plus, they're all guaranteed to be divinely delicious, gluten free, and vegan!

In the back of the book, we've included a glossary filled with the definitions sprinkled throughout the book as well as some other technique, item, and equipment terms. Finally, we share some wonderful resources you can use to further your gluten-free vegan journey.

Extras

Throughout the book, you'll find sidebars, there to guide you along and offer additional information.

DEFINITION

These mini-dictionaries define terms, ingredients, and techniques you may not be familiar with.

MEATLESS AND WHEATLESS

These helpful hints expound upon certain facts and ideas presented in the text.

AGAINST THE GRAIN

Be sure to heed the warnings shared in this sidebar.

CORNUCOPIA

Read these sidebars for some fun, miscellaneous ideas and related reflections.

Plant-Based Dietitian Recommends: Being a gluten-free vegan can be challenging enough all on its own. Because some of you may be transitioning your diet to include healthier choices, we've included many recipes in this book that are oil free. On the flip side, for those who are taking a moderation approach, we've also included recipes that contain nonhydrogenated margarine or various types of oils, refined vegan sweeteners, and a couple other processed foods. To include everyone, we've added "Plant-Based Dietitian Recommends" notes throughout recipes containing those ingredients. Julieanna, your plant-based dietitian, is looking out for your optimal health choices and provides you with alternatives to keep your diet 100 percent whole foods. If you have any chronic health conditions or are trying to lose weight, we advise you to follow these suggestions.

Acknowledgments

We would like to thank several people for all their help and assistance in writing this book: Tom Stevens, Christy Wagner, Marie Butler-Knight, and the rest of the Alpha Books team who helped bring this book to fruition. Much appreciation to Marilyn Allen and her team at Allen O'Shea Literary Agency.

Thanks, too, to our fellow *VegNews* columnist, vegan author, photographer, and blogger extraordinaire, Hannah Kaminsky, for graciously agreeing to do the food styling and photo for the cover of this book.

Beverly would like to thank her friends and family for all their love and support during the writing of this book. She also wants to thank her cat companion, Luna, for the many hours of snuggling and purring on her lap while sitting at the computer typing out her recipes. And most of all, she would like to thank Ray Sammartano, her partner in life as well as co-author on her two previous *Complete Idiot's Guides*, for his support, helpful suggestions, and insights regarding content, and for being her chief taste-tester through culinary successes and almost-successes.

Julieanna would like to thank her husband, Aviv, and little ones, Maya and Ben, for their ceaseless support and patience. She also has limitless appreciation for the sustenance and backbone of her family and friends while working on this book, especially her mom and dad, Renee, Rachel, Dina, and Jesse.

And lastly, we would like to thank all the other dedicated vegan writers, cookbook authors, activists, and other folks out there who are dedicated to spreading the vegan message and who strive to improve their own lives as well as the lives of the many creatures we share this planet with.

Trademarks

All terms mentioned in this book that are known to be or are suspected of being trademarks or service marks have been appropriately capitalized. Alpha Books and Penguin Group (USA) Inc. cannot attest to the accuracy of this information. Use of a term in this book should not be regarded as affecting the validity of any trademark or service mark.

Living Gluten Free and Vegan

An increase in incidence of gluten-intolerance, food allergies, and celiac disease in recent years is impossible to deny. In Chapter 1, we explain the difference between each of these issues and how you can determine which you may be experiencing—if you haven't already. We walk you through which ingredients and foods you need to avoid so you can keep your body feeling fantastic and symptom free. We also offer ample details to help you approach the vast array of gluten-free options available to you.

Whether you're a well-seasoned vegan or a fresh and curious newbie, Chapter 1 provides you with a hearty helping of facts and figures explaining the many health benefits a gluten-free vegan diet offers. We give you a breakdown of the most health-promoting diet, including a detailed description of the Plant-Based Food Guide Pyramid. With this information, you'll be ready to prevent and reverse disease, and achieve and maintain your ideal body weight effortlessly.

In Chapter 2, we help you set up your kitchen for gluten-free vegan-cooking freedom. From appliances to gadgets and food to fill your pantry, fridge, and freezer, you'll be ready to create delicious, nutritious, gluten-free vegan meals whenever the mood strikes.

Finally, Chapter 3 tops off your preparation needs by delving into substitutions and replacements for gluten-containing or animal-based items now on the "do not use" list.

The Gluten-Free Vegan

In This Chapter

- A look at gluten intolerance
- Finding gluten where it hides
- The benefits of a vegan lifestyle
- Whole foods = whole health

Whether you were vegan first and then went gluten free or vice versa, you might feel a bit limited in your cuisine options. You're not alone. The combined gluten-free vegan population is booming with new members, many of them wondering what's left to eat.

In this chapter, we explore this delicious, health-promoting, Earth-loving, compassionate way of life and show you some of the many wonderful things you *can* still eat.

What's the Big Deal About Gluten?

Plenty, as you well know if you or a loved one has a gluten sensitivity, intolerance, or allergy. Although difficult to diagnose and commonly missed, the number of cases of gluten sensitivity has increased in recent years. Once considered rare, celiac disease (also known as celiac sprue) has become common.

Fortunately for those suffering with gluten issues, the food industry has taken notice and responded with a flood of gluten-free products. Even entire stores—online as well as brick-and-mortar—are dedicated to gluten-free goods. Some factories and restaurants devote specific kitchens—or entire buildings—to prevent cross-contamination of gluten in their products.

What Is Gluten?

All this talk about gluten has caused quite a stir. But what is gluten? Gluten is a protein found in wheat and other cereal grains, including rye, barley, and sometimes oats. When you wash away all the starch from these cereal flours, the water-insoluble gluten remains.

The main difference between having an intolerance, allergy, or celiac disease is the severity of the repercussions if gluten is consumed. People with sensitivities respond differently to gluten. Some can be symptom free with a small dose while others can suffer massively. You may have a mild intolerance when you consume it, manifesting as some gastrointestinal (GI) discomfort, fatigue, or eczema. Or on the extreme side of the spectrum, if you have celiac disease, you may become asthmatic when inhaling gluten-containing flour or damage your GI tract simply by consuming it. While an intolerance can make you miserable, a true food allergy can be more dangerous, especially when a severe allergic reaction is possible.

CORNUCOPIA

You can be allergic to wheat for a reason other than the gluten component. Sometimes it's one of the other proteins in wheat causing the allergy. In addition to gluten, wheat also contains albumin, globulin, and gliadin. So you may be able to eat barley, rye, and oats without any problem but have to omit all wheat products.

No cure yet exists for celiac disease. Whether you have a mild intolerance to gluten or full-fledged celiac disease, avoiding gluten protein is your best bet. With a bit of finesse and some careful investigating—and the mouthwatering recipes you'll find in this book—you can be cleared of your symptoms and restored to optimum health. Living a gluten-free life will stop any symptoms and allow the intestines to heal within 3 to 6 months for children, and 2 or 3 years for adults.

To learn more about the basics of living gluten free, check out *The Complete Idiot's Guide to Gluten-Free Eating* (Alpha Books, 2007).

Tips for Dealing with Celiac Disease

Regardless of the origin of your gluten intolerance, the only treatment is to refrain from eating any gluten-containing ingredients. In addition, you can try a few tricks to help promote gut health:

- Avoid overusing antibiotics. They destroy healthful bacteria in the intestines, leaving room for harmful bacteria and yeast to grow.

- Eliminate processed sugar and products containing sugar. They cause inflammation and feed yeasts in the gut.

- If possible, get tested for other food allergies, intolerances, or sensitivities. *Cross-reactivity* commonly accompanies gluten sensitivity. Common cross-reactive associations with gluten include dairy, nightshade vegetables, and carageenan.

- Consider taking *probiotics* to support healthy flora in your gut. Probiotics can be found in vegan yogurts and fermented foods like miso, sauerkraut, and tempeh. However, they may be best taken via supplement to ensure a large enough dose to be effective.

DEFINITION

Cross-reactivity is a condition where your body's immune system mistakes other food proteins for ones you can't tolerate and creates an autoimmune reaction to them, making you react to these other foods in the same way as with gluten. **Probiotics** are live microorganisms that, when consumed in adequate quantities, improve immunity and digestion.

The Gluten Detective

Gluten (Latin for "glue") has several functions in cooking. It adds a sticky texture to foods, provides elasticity, promotes volume in bread products, contributes to thickness, and can be made to resemble animal protein for the creation of a wide variety of mock meats.

Because gluten is so functional, food manufacturers use it quite often, making it tough to avoid. You need to be cautious and well versed in gluten jargon to avoid accidentally consuming the enemy.

Deciphering Food Labels

Gluten-containing ingredients go by a wide variety of names. Beyond whole grains, gluten is found in all products containing these grains or their derivatives: barley, einkorn, emmer (a hard, red wheat), farro, kamut, oats (unless they're specified as gluten free), rye, spelt, triticale, and wheat (cracked wheat, wheat bran, wheat starch, wheat germ).

Wheat is especially popular in the food industry because it can be converted and used in millions of products. The intact grain can be manufactured into flours, starches, proteins, thickeners, fillers, and more.

Be wary when you see the following ingredients and products on ingredient lists or menus:

All-purpose flour

Baked goods

Baking powder

Battered foods

Bromated flour

Burgers (veggie burgers, too)

Bouillon cubes

Bran

Bread

Breadcrumbs

Brown rice syrup (unless specified gluten free)

Candy

Cereal

Cereal extract

Chips/potato chips

Cornbread

Couscous

Cracker meal

Crackers

Croquettes

Dextrin

Durum

Durum flour

Enriched flour

Farina

Flour

French fries

Gluten

Graham flour

Grain coffee substitute

Granola

Gravies

Hydrolyzed plant protein

Hydrolyzed vegetable protein

Icings

Imitation fish

Instant cocoa

Luncheon meats

Maltodextrin

Matzo

Meatloaf or meatballs (veggie, too)

Modified food starch

Ovaltine

Pâté

Phosphated flour

Piecrusts

Postum

Processed meats

Rice mixes

Salad dressings

Sauces

Sausages

Seasonings

Self-rising flour

Semolina

Soy sauce

Stabilizers

Stuffing

Surimi

Tamari (unless specified wheat free)

Tempura

Xanthan gum

Gluten can also be present in nonfood items like medications, supplements, and lip balm, so read labels very carefully. Over time your detective skills will sharpen and knowing what to avoid will become second nature.

Gluten-Free Options

Gluten free doesn't mean grain free, and plenty of delicious grain-based options are waiting for you at your local market. You just have to know what to look for. Never before has there been such a vast array of gluten-free products as there is today. Pastas, breads, tortillas, pizzas, cakes, piecrusts, and everything you could ever miss on a gluten-free diet is readily available in gluten-free versions.

Gluten-free grains and other foods that are safe for your consumption include amaranth, arrowroot, buckwheat, cassava, corn, flax, montina (Indian rice grass), Job's tears, kasha, legumes (all beans, peas, and lentils—like black bean, chickpea, fava and garfava bean, green pea, pinto bean, and soy—either in their whole form or ground into flours), millet, nuts, potatoes, quinoa, rice, sago, seeds, sorghum, tapioca, taro, teff, wild rice, and yucca.

Depending on where you live, most of these products should be on your grocer's shelves. Even if they're not, you can still have anything you desire delivered to your door with a click of the mouse from any of the multitude of gluten-free online stores. (We've listed a bunch in Appendix B.)

Living Vegan

Veganism is not merely a growing trend. Rather, it's a lifestyle choice that's growing in popularity as more people become aware of the health benefits of eating a plant-based, animal-free diet. According to a recent poll approximately 1.4 percent of the U.S. population is currently vegan, and as a result, information about vegan restaurants and foods is popping up nearly everywhere you look.

Vegans typically don't eat any type of animal flesh (red meat, chicken, turkey, pork, fish, etc.), dairy products, eggs, gelatin, or honey. They abstain from wearing clothing or items made with animal products, including fur, leather, silk, wool, feathers, or pearls. They also avoid anything made with animal-based ingredients such as cosmetics, toiletries, or household goods.

For Your Health

Experts have known for centuries that the more whole-plant foods you eat, the healthier you're likely to be. Consider Hippocrates's profound declaration made approximately 2,400 years ago: "Let thy food be thy medicine, and thy medicine be thy food." Scientists have been gathering compelling data ever since.

It's impossible to argue with the massive amounts of research confirming how potent vegetables, fruits, whole grains, legumes, nuts, and seeds are for your body. Each of these food groups are overflowing with *phytonutrients*, *antioxidants*, vitamins, minerals, fiber, and water.

> **DEFINITION**
>
> **Phytonutrients** are naturally occurring compounds in plants that contain numerous health benefits, including performing antioxidant, anti-inflammatory, antiseptic, and a host of other activities. **Antioxidants** are certain vitamins, minerals, and phytonutrients that slow or stop the process of oxidation, which is what leads to aging and chronic disease development.

A plant-based diet is good for you in two ways: it eliminates the components of a standard diet that promote disease and it provides nourishment in the doses your body requires. You can get everything you need to fight illness, ensure loads of energy, and feel great without the burden of calculating calories and fat grams, or the worry of constantly popping supplements.

As Nature Intended

Mother Nature has it all down perfectly. Everything from the earth packs a nutritional punch and empowers your body to be its best. Nutrients you need come in the right ratios and are easily assimilated into your cells when you eat whole, intact foods. So why reinvent the wheel?

Unfortunately these days, many foods that have become staples on most people's plates are so far removed from their original packaging they're nearly unrecognizable. The "foods" have traveled such a long journey down the processing conveyer belt, much of the beneficial fiber, vitamins, and minerals have been stripped away and replaced by other nonfood items, perhaps along with some synthetic vitamins and minerals. Ultimately, you end up with a nonfood item dressed up as a food.

Why are we so inundated with processed foods? Because that's the way the food industry wants it. Researchers for companies that make fast and processed foods have determined the precise combination of sweet, salty, and fatty your taste buds require to keep you coming back for more and more of their products. This promotes cravings and a vicious cycle of dependence.

However, there's a pot of gold waiting at the end of the rainbow of whole, plant foods. Eliminating the addictive sugary, salty, and fatty "un-foods" from your diet and honing in on delicious, satisfying whole foods—like the ones you'll find recipes for in this book—will release your taste buds and brain chemistry from the grip of that cycle and unleash the wide-ranging flavors of nature's bounty.

A Whole New Pyramid

The Plant-Based Food Guide Pyramid provides a guideline for structuring your daily food intake. The goal is to base your diet primarily on foods from the bottom of the pyramid and include lesser amounts of the foods as you work your way up. Items listed at the top of the pyramid are to be included the least.

Unlike the USDA's version of the food pyramid, fruits and vegetables serve as the base in the plant-based version, right above drinking adequate fluids and performing exercise on a daily basis. Any and all fruits and vegetables are included here because they serve as nutrient powerhouses, providing ample amounts of *carotenoids*, vitamins A and C, folate, potassium, carbohydrates, water, and fiber.

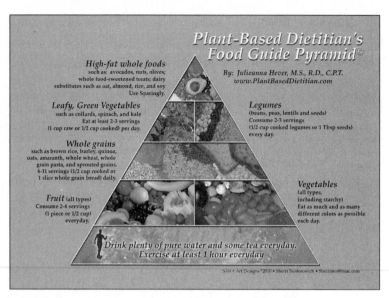

The Plant-Based Food Guide Pyramid provides a guideline for getting the whole, plant-based foods you need every day.

DEFINITION

Carotenoids are a category of up to hundreds of naturally occurring organic pigments in plants with red, orange, and yellow hues, several of which have potent antioxidant properties.

Because leafy greens have their own category, some vegetables to emphasize on the base include mushrooms, carrots, cauliflower, peppers, beets, cucumbers, squash, eggplant, garlic, onions, green beans, snap peas, potatoes, yams, corn, fennel, fresh herbs, and celery.

Next up, carbohydrate-rich whole grains. Excellent sources of energy, whole grains provide fiber, protein, iron, selenium, manganese, magnesium, and B vitamins. When living gluten free, this is the category most affected. To get the vitamins and minerals whole grains provide, but still avoid gluten, load up your plate with quinoa, corn, amaranth, millet, brown rice, sorghum, buckwheat, wild rice, and teff.

Leafy greens—like kale, collard greens, dandelion greens, spinach, beet greens, turnip greens, lettuce, bok choy, Swiss chard, rainbow chard, brussels sprouts, sea vegetables, broccoli, and cabbage—get their very own category because they really are special. Brimming with nutrients like calcium; fiber; folate; iron; magnesium;

manganese; potassium; riboflavin, vitamins K, A, C, B$_6$, and E; and phytochemicals such as lutein, beta-cryptoxanthin, zeaxanthin, and beta-carotene, leafy greens deserve some extra attention in your diet.

Next-door neighbors to the leafy greens are health-boosting legumes. Looking for hearty sources of protein, fiber, folate, thiamine, iron, calcium, magnesium, zinc, and potassium? Legumes are the answer. Indulge in a vast variety of available beans, lentils, peas, and soy products (edamame, tempeh, and tofu) to get your daily dose.

Seeds are also included in the legumes section because you need small quantities of them (approximately 1 or 2 tablespoons) daily to get your omega-3 fatty acids. Choose from flax, hemp, or chia seeds for optimal fat profiles. Sesame seeds add a mega dose of calcium, which is a welcomed bonus.

Finally, at the peak of the pyramid, you'll find high-fat whole foods, fortified non-dairy substitutes, and whole food–sweetened treats. Avocados, nuts, and olives are excellent sources of fat and vitamin E. Fortified plant milks can be an easy way to get your daily dose of vitamins D and B$_{12}$. Be sure to choose unsweetened versions to avoid added sugars, and use all items from this category sparingly.

AGAINST THE GRAIN

If weight loss is your goal, minimize the fatty and sugary choices as much as possible because these foods are likely to keep on the pounds.

To learn more about the vegan lifestyle, please pick up a copy of *The Complete Idiot's Guide to Vegan Living* (Alpha Books, 2005) and *The Complete Idiot's Guide to Vegan Cooking* (Alpha Books, 2008), written by co-author Beverly along with Ray Sammartano.

Nutritional Necessities

To fight disease, support immune function, maintain an ideal weight, and perform optimally, your body needs a certain amount of macronutrients (carbohydrate, protein, and fat) and micronutrients (vitamins and minerals). Fantastically, whole-plant foods provide everything in perfect quantity, save for one or two vitamins. Just by eating a whole vegan diet puts you ahead of the game, even if it's gluten free.

Mini Macro Review

A combination of three macronutrients—carbohydrate (a.k.a. carbs), protein, and fat—are the major components that make up your food and is where you derive all your calories from. These life-sustaining constituents are necessary for energy, growth, and development. The vast majority of your diet should come from carbs, as seen earlier in the pyramid. Foods primarily composed of carbohydrates include vegetables, fruits, whole grains, and legumes. Carbs are converted into glucose the quickest and are the sole source of energy your brain uses.

You can categorize carbs into simple and complex. Simple carbs are absorbed more readily into the bloodstream, providing near-instant energy. Whole, vegan food sources high in simple carbs include fruits (especially dried), maple syrup, and brown rice syrup.

Complex carbs are lengthier-chained molecules that are further divided into starches and fibers. Starches are absorbable; provide longer-lasting energy than simple carbs; and can be found in potatoes, peas, corn, root vegetables, and whole grains. Unlike starch, fiber is not digestible or usable for energy. Separated into either soluble or insoluble, fibers include plant parts that boost health in a multitude of ways. Soluble fibers help lower blood cholesterol levels and are found in oats, beans, peas, apples, citrus fruits, and carrots. Insoluble fibers—found in fibrous vegetables, whole grains, and nuts—moderate blood sugar levels, aid weight loss, remove excess hormones and heavy metals from the blood, and prevent colorectal cancer.

AGAINST THE GRAIN

Most oat-based products contain traces of gluten due to oat crops being grown so close to wheat crops or as a result of using shared milling facilities. However, uncontaminated, gluten-free versions are now available. Most people with celiac disease can tolerate these oats with a small exception of those sensitive to a compound called avenin.

Protein plays a vital role in pretty much every structure and function of the human body. It makes up your nails, hair, muscles, and skin as well as enzymes, hormones, blood, and immune cells. Composed from different arrangements of 20 amino acids, proteins constantly are broken down and rebuilt in your body as necessary. Out of those 20 amino acids, only 9 must be taken in from the diet and are, therefore, considered essential. It's virtually impossible *not* to get adequate amounts of protein on an unrefined, vegan diet. Even a banana—considered a starchy carb—contains 5 percent of its calories from protein. Brown rice has 9 percent, and leafy greens contain up to half of their total calories from protein. Lentils, beans, and soy products are loaded with more than enough protein to meet your daily quota.

Completing the macronutrient triad is fat. Dietary fat is a concentrated source of energy and is important for helping absorb fat-soluble vitamins; providing essential fatty acids; and contributing to coagulation, gene expression, and inflammation. You really don't need much fat in your diet and, like carbs and protein, fat is ubiquitous in the plant-based world. Most people consume too much fat, which has been shown to contribute to the development and progression of chronic disease. Further, the type of fat you consume is as important—if not more so—than how much.

First, some fatty acid terminology:

Saturated fat is mostly found in animal products, but also in the plant world from tropical oils like coconut, palm, and palm kernel oil. It's completely unnecessary in the diet.

Trans fat, possibly worse for your health than saturated fat, is created via a process called hydrogenation and is used to extend the shelf life of processed or fried foods.

Omega-3 fatty acids are a family of essential polyunsaturated fats (ALA, EPA, and DHA) found in flaxseeds, hemp seeds, chia seeds, soybeans, tofu, leafy green vegetables, and walnuts. They are anti-inflammatory, enhance your immune system, and help protect your heart.

Alpha-linolenic acid (ALA) is an omega-3 fatty acid found in plants (chiefly in seed oils) that ultimately can be converted into EPA and then DHA.

Omega-6 fatty acids are a group of essential polyunsaturated fats widely available in many dietary sources, especially vegetable oils.

Saturated and trans fats contribute to cancer, heart disease, and kidney disease and interfere with liver function and essential fatty acid metabolism, so avoid them as much as possible. You do, however, need essential fatty acids because your body cannot produce these on its own.

As a herbivore, you don't have a direct source for the two indispensable long-chain omega-3 fatty acids EPA and DHA. Your body makes these via the conversion of alpha-linolenic acid. To achieve a proper fatty acid balance, eat the majority of your fat from flaxseeds, hemp seeds, chia seeds, leafy green vegetables, soy products (soybeans and tofu), and walnuts. Also, limit your intake of trans fatty acids (found in snack foods, fried foods, fast foods, and commercially baked goods). Finally, moderate your consumption of omega-6 fatty acids, especially from vegetable oils.

Getting the Vitamins and Minerals You Need

Vitamins and minerals are micronutrients essential in small amounts for survival. Think of them as little helpers that enable all your body's functions to take place. From blood clotting and bone development to food metabolism and building genetic material, vitamins and minerals are very busy and absolutely critical. Most of these compounds are plentiful in plant foods. The only exceptions are vitamins B_{12} and D.

Vitamin B_{12}, also known as cobalamin, is synthesized by microorganisms. Animals consume these microorganisms along with the dirt remaining on their plant cuisine, making B_{12} present in their meat. So if you like to eat your produce washed, rinsed, and dirt free, you need to supplement your herbivorous diet with the vitamin. Vitamin B_{12} is involved in nerve function, red blood cell production, and DNA formation. Having barriers to absorption is not uncommon, and you usually don't know you're deficient in vitamin B_{12} until it's too late. Be proactive and mind your B! You need about 5 to 10 micrograms per day, which you can find in a supplement or in fortified plant milks and nutritional yeast.

Vitamin D, the sunshine vitamin, is a hot topic these days. Although no plant sources of vitamin D exist, you can create it in your body when you expose your skin to sunlight. Recent research suggests that many chronic diseases are associated with vitamin D deficiency, including many cancers, osteoporosis, autoimmune disease, diabetes, and heart disease. Because there's currently a worldwide vitamin D deficiency, a vegan diet can't be singled out as the cause. Researchers are questioning the reasons why and how, as well as trying to determine the ideal protocol for preventing and reversing deficiency.

Current recommendations are to regularly monitor your blood level of 25-hydroxyvitamin D. If you don't have a level above 35 to 40 ng/mL, try exposing as much of your skin as possible without sunscreen (except on your face) 3 to 5 days a week during peak hours (10 A.M. to 2 P.M.) for about 10 to 15 minutes, depending on your skin color. If this doesn't work and your levels remain low, take a vitamin D_2 (vegan) supplement for a few months and recheck your blood level.

We could fill a whole book on vegan nutrition—and Julieanna has! For everything you need to know about whole-food, plant-based, vegan nutrition, look to *The Complete Idiot's Guide to Plant-Based Nutrition* (Alpha Books, 2011).

When you take time and think before you make a food choice, you gain a special awareness about what you're really eating. We think that's a blessing in disguise. Many people sail through life eating either out of convenience or food preference. But you now have the opportunity to redefine eating as nourishment for your body, your temple. Choosing a vegan lifestyle is based on making choices out of compassion. Add a food intolerance into the mix, and now you're using mind, body, and spirit to make appropriate food decisions. You'll benefit in so many areas by doing so.

The Least You Need to Know

- Diagnosing gluten intolerance, allergy, or celiac disease will help you find the foods that *do* work for you.
- Gluten hides behind many different aliases. Expand your gluten vocabulary to be sure you can completely avoid it and all its forms.
- All essential nutrients can be found abundantly in whole-plant foods, except vitamins B_{12} and D. You can supplement B_{12} with fortified foods or a pill and get D from the sun or supplements, if necessary.

The Perfectly Prepped Kitchen

In This Chapter

- Handy appliances and tools
- Essential equipment to have on hand
- Stocking your gluten-free vegan pantry

One of the first steps to success for gluten-free vegan cooking is having a well-stocked kitchen. After all, if you have everything you need at hand, preparing delicious dishes will be a snap. Keeping your pantry, fridge, and freezer stocked and loaded will enable you to whip up a masterpiece at a moment's inspiration. With a bunch of staples and perhaps a few afterthoughts, dinner can be on the table in no time!

What's more, gluten-free vegan cooking does not require any special tools or advanced culinary techniques. Simplicity is key, and we show you exactly how to discover and implement basic methods in your preparation.

Tools of the Gluten-Free Vegan Trade

Begin by performing a quick scan of your kitchen's inventory to see what you already have. You can always make do with what's easily accessible and then start thinking about saving for certain items you'd like to eventually add to your repertoire. There's a wide spectrum, from simple to extraordinary, when it comes to kitchen equipment, so choose according to your needs and preferences.

AGAINST THE GRAIN

Cross-contamination of gluten-containing ingredients can be an issue in a kitchen shared with gluten eaters. Depending on your level of sensitivity, consider keeping a set of separate cookware, dishes, bowls, and utensils to prevent accidental gluten consumption.

Applicable Appliances

As in basic cooking, a stovetop and oven are helpful (unless you're on a 100 percent raw diet). Two other critical components to keep nearby are a good blender and a food processor. These two appliances perform what human hands aren't capable of, and you'll use them both at least once a day.

Your food processor is perfect for fine chopping, puréeing, and blending while maintaining some texture. You also can slice, dice, shred, and julienne with the various blades that come with it. Choose full blast or pulse for chunkier pieces. You can even make nut butter, gluten-free flours, salsas, spreads, sauces, and dips.

You can get away with less, price-wise, on the food processor, but ultimately, you get what you pay for, especially in terms of a blender. The high-powered machines are unmatched in their ability to completely liquefy anything. They're great for making green smoothies and sauces. You can even make a soup directly in the high-powered blender because the blades rotate so fast, the resulting friction heats up the contents after a couple minutes!

An immersion blender, a handheld sticklike blender, is great for puréeing soups directly in the pot. This reduces the chances for splash-induced burns when transferring soup from pot to blender and back.

If you like raw cuisine (and we share some delicious raw recipes later in the book), you may want to invest in a dehydrator. These handy machines enable you to dehydrate vegetables, fruits, and other items at a temperature that maintains the standards for raw (less than 118°F). Kale chips, crackers, and other healthful gourmet treats are all easy with a dehydrator.

Rice cookers/steamers are another helpful appliance to have available. Instead of worrying about burning your grains, you can comfortably add the right ratio of grains to water, push start, and enjoy perfectly cooked steamed grains when you hear the beep. Plus, rice cookers warm your food until you turn it off, so you can have brown rice, quinoa, and more at your disposal all day long. You can even steam your veggies in these simple-to-use cookers.

Other Helpful Tools and Equipment

Choosing the appropriate cookware, utensils, and other useful tools will simplify and expedite your prep work, improve your finished dishes, and keep you motivated to get creative in the kitchen.

When it comes to cookware, you need a good set of stainless steel, cast iron, or clay pots and pans that promote even cooking, are easy to wash, and are durable and sturdy. Don't automatically reach for the nonstick pans. Research has shown nonstick cookware may be harmful to your health. At high temperatures, and when scratched by utensils, the chemicals are released into the food and are carcinogenic (cancer-promoting). Fortunately, you don't need nonstick for your food to not stick. A mere bit of attention to your food during cooking, keeping it moist and moving around, will prevent sticking.

Recently, new lines of nontoxic nonstick cookware using safe technology approved by the FDA have come to market. They're getting rave reviews by people using the products and exhibit exceptional nonstick performance. Companies like SafePan and Cuisinart are replacing the petroleum-based products with ceramic for eco-friendly, healthy options. Whenever you see the word *nonstick* in this book, we are referring to these products. Of course, you can also substitute the other nontoxic types of cookware mentioned in our recipes.

We recommend silicone bakeware. As an inert compound, it won't leech into your food, emit fumes, or pose health risks. It's naturally nonstick, tolerates heat and cold well, and comes in every shape and size.

With other essential tools—such as measuring cups, bowls, colanders, steamer baskets, cutting boards, spoons, spatulas, ladles, whisks, and tongs—stick with stainless steel, glass, wood, bamboo, or silicone, and try to limit your use of plastic and aluminum-based materials, which migrate into the food it has contact with. Associations have been found between several plastics used in food packaging and plastic wrap with cancers, hormonal changes, impaired immunity, and liver dysfunction, among other problems. Aluminum has been shown to contribute to damage to the nervous system, dementia, memory loss, and Alzheimer's disease.

All veggie lovers need a good set of knives for chopping, slicing, and dicing. Opt for a set that includes at least a chef's knife, a long serrated knife, and a paring knife because these are the most frequently used. Select knives that are comfortable in your hand and easy to sharpen.

Here are some other fun gadgets to consider adding to your collection:

- Zester or grater or Microplane to zest citrus, hand-shred veggies, easily mince ginger or garlic, and grate nutmeg.

- Assorted sizes of ice cream scoops for perfectly portioning equal sizes and easily filling muffin cups.

- Spiral slicer (a.k.a. spiralizer) to make raw ribbons or noodles out of zucchini, daikon radish, cucumber, squash, carrot, and sweet potato.

- Garlic press to intensify garlic flavor and its dispersal throughout your dish.

- Wooden citrus reamer or citrus press to extract the most juice from citrus.

Stocked and Loaded

Now that you're equipped and ready to go, all you need are the ingredients to create culinary magic. Stock your pantry, fridge, and freezer with some savvy essentials and keep them refreshed. It's essential to have yummy ingredients so you can always make healthy choices at a growling stomach's first alert.

Remember that you don't *have* to have everything we list here. Think of these as your grand shopping lists, so you can make every recipe in this book and still have leftovers. Of course, most people don't shop that way. Whether you shop once, twice, or more per week, be sure to keep your produce fresh. This may mean a quick trip to the farmers' market between store trips or belonging to a CSA (Community Supported Agriculture) where you can pick up freshly plucked produce weekly from your local farm or even have it delivered to your door.

CORNUCOPIA

For more information on finding a CSA near you, visit Local Harvest's website at localharvest.org/csa.

The Vegified Pantry

In the pantry, stock up on assorted gluten-free whole grains such as amaranth, brown rice, buckwheat, oats, quinoa, wild rice, and black forbidden rice. Intact whole grains don't last as long as pearled or hulled grains because the bran and germ portions of the grain—the parts that are removed when refined—go rancid quicker than the other portions due to their higher fat content. In your cool, dark pantry, you can store whole grains for several months at a time. Be sure to keep them in a tightly sealed package. In warmer temperatures, store your grains in the refrigerator.

Also keep on hand products made with gluten-free grains such as corn, brown rice, or hemp tortillas; pastas made from corn, soy, quinoa, amaranth, artichoke, and brown rice; and gluten-free whole-grain breads, crackers, rice cakes, and corn thins.

For baking purposes, stock up on these gluten-free whole-grain flours and other baking ingredients: gluten-free all-purpose baking flour, brown rice flour or flakes, quinoa flour or flakes, millet flour, sorghum flour, cornmeal, cornstarch, potato starch, tapioca starch, Ener-G Egg Replacer, agar powder or agar-agar, arrowroot, gluten-free baking powder, baking soda, cream of tartar, guar gum, gluten-free xanthan gum, rapid-rise active yeast, and salt. You can also grab some other gluten-free flours such as black bean, chickpea, garfava bean, almond meal, and gluten-free oat if you prefer.

Legumes are a pantry essential. These little packages of goodness are bursting with high-quality nutrition. Dried beans of any and every variety, peas, and lentils can be stored in a cool, dry place like your pantry for about a year. Peanuts (yep, a legume) last about 9 months. Canned beans can hang out for about 2 years before expiring, but be sure to check the "best by" date. Keep a stash of chickpeas, black beans, pinto beans, kidney beans, red beans, black-eyed peas, green and yellow split peas, lentils, red lentils, cannellini (or white kidney) beans, adzuki (or aduki) beans, navy beans, and soy beans. Tons of different varieties of legumes are available and waiting to be experimented with—and we recommend you do! When purchasing canned beans, opt for salt-free and BPA-free selections if available.

MEATLESS AND WHEATLESS

Keep a box of iodized salt on hand. In addition to a dietary source of iodine, the salt has other functions in baking than just flavoring. You can also purchase some Himalayan pink or Celtic sea salt. We like to use it in our recipes as a flavoring agent.

Here are some other pantry items to stock up on:

- Aseptic plant-based almond, soy, hemp, oat, and rice milks (Store in the fridge after opening.)

- Sea vegetables such as nori, kombu, wakame, dulse, and kelp

- Canned artichoke hearts (packed in water), corn, olives, roasted red peppers (packed in water), water chestnuts, puréed pumpkin, and sweet potato

- Canned tomatoes (whole, crushed, diced, and fire-roasted varieties), tomato paste, tomato sauce, and sun-dried tomatoes

- Raw nut butters or seed butters like tahini (Refrigerate after opening.)

- Dried dates, raisins, apricots, prunes, cranberries, and cherries

- Hot pepper sauces and salsas

- Balsamic, red wine, brown rice, rice wine, apple cider, and other vinegars

- Blackstrap molasses, sorghum syrup, gluten-free brown rice syrup, and 100 percent pure maple syrup

- Cold-pressed extra-virgin olive oil and expeller-pressed toasted sesame oil and sunflower oil

- Raw cacao nibs, raw cacao powder, cocoa powder, and vegan chocolate chips or bars

In Cold Storage and in Plain Sight

As a gluten-free vegan, much of your food choices are fresh and fabulous. So clear off your countertops and make room in the fridge.

Fresh fruits and veggies don't last very long because they're alive with nutrients— which is part of the reason they're so excellent for your body. So you need to replenish your stores regularly and consistently. Rainbows of color constantly in your range of view will encourage and remind you to make good selections. Having fresh fruits, prepped salads and soups, and other colorful munchies ready to eat enables you to grab healthful foods at the first sign of hunger.

Certain fresh fruits and veggies should live, temporarily, on your countertops. Store your apples, citrus, bananas, avocados, peaches, plums, nectarines, garlic, tomatoes, and seasonal fruits like persimmons and cherimoyas in plain sight on the counter so they're always ready to go.

Onions, shallots, garlic, potatoes, sweet potatoes, and yams are best stored in cool, dark, well-ventilated places, so find a place in your pantry to stash these staples. Root vegetables like beets, turnips, parsnips, celeriac, rutabagas, and radishes are best stored in perforated bags in the crisper drawer of the refrigerator.

When choosing nuts and seeds, opt for raw and organic whenever possible. To ensure your omega-3 fatty acid intake and to make flax eggs and other recipes, keep flax-seeds on hand, too. You can buy whole flaxseeds if you plan to grind them before use or buy ground flaxseeds. Store these in your fridge.

Also in your refrigerator, you can store …

- Plant-based almond, soy, hemp, oat, and rice milks (These come refriger-ated as well as shelf-stable until opened; choose according to your taste preference.)

- Whole-fruit jams and some fruits—especially tomatoes and berries

- Fresh dill, rosemary, basil, cilantro, parsley, and other herbs

- Raw leafy greens, carrots, broccoli, cauliflower, cabbage, lettuce, radishes, turnips, zucchini, squash, and other fresh vegetables

- Silken, firm, extra-firm, and super firm tofu for use in recipes and gluten-free tempeh

- Jars of minced garlic and ginger for emergencies when you run out of the fresh varieties

- Flax, hemp, chia, sunflower, pumpkin, and sesame seeds, along with almonds, cashews, peanuts, pecans, and walnuts

- Dijon and spicy brown mustard, ketchup, and prepared horseradish, plus pure kosher dill pickles and pickle relish (without sugar or preservatives)

Your freezer can be home to lots of happy helpers. Frozen fruits and veggies, both plain and mixed blends, can speed up your cooking and food prep exponentially. Not having to wash and chop can save many minutes. Plus, frozen goods last for up to a year, so you can stock up and always have ready-to-use options.

MEATLESS AND WHEATLESS

Save room in your freezer for leftovers. It simplifies your life to make your meals in larger portions and then freeze the extras for later.

When stocking your freezer, choose frozen peeled bananas and any other fruits (organic, if possible), including berries, pineapple, mango, and peaches. For frozen veggies, buy frozen cut corn, peas, edamame, greens, broccoli, mushrooms, mixed vegetable blends, and other vegetables. Other good options include precooked brown rice, whole-fruit popsicles or sorbet, and nondairy ice cream.

Souped-Up Spice Rack

Spice is, well, the spice of life! You can transform any food from *blah* to *wow* with the right seasonings. It's easy to be intimidated by the vast array of dried herbs and spices on the grocery shelves, but you needn't be. You know your palate better than anyone and can experiment to find just what you like. Practicing with recipes helps you learn which combinations work and don't work for you. Then adjust accordingly.

An essential collection of dried herbs and spices could include gomasio, sea veggie shakers, allspice, anise, basil, cardamom, cayenne, chili powder, ground chipotle powder, ground cinnamon, ground cloves, ground coriander, ground cumin, curry powder, dill weed, fennel seeds or ground fennel, garlic powder or garlic granules, ground ginger, lemongrass, ground mace, marjoram, dried mustard, whole nutmeg, onion powder, oregano, smoked or sweet paprika, black pepper or peppercorns, crushed red pepper flakes, rosemary, rubbed sage, star anise, thyme, turmeric, and wasabi powder.

And don't forget your blends! You can find blends to match any mood, any culture, and every taste bud. Try garam masala, Cajun seasoning blend, Chinese five-spice powder, Jamaican jerk seasoning, herbes de Provence, and zahtar for a party of flavors.

The Least You Need to Know

- You don't need any fancy equipment for gluten-free vegan cooking; a good blender, food processor, stove, set of knives, some basic cooking utensils and gadgets, and some pots and pans are plenty to start with.
- Keep your pantry stocked with gluten-free whole grains, legumes, and various spices, and your countertop abundant with fresh produce.
- Your fridge should be bursting with colorful fruits, veggies, nuts, seeds, condiments, and some whole soy options.
- Store frozen produce and leftovers in your freezer to boost longevity and increase efficiency.

Savvy Substitutions

In This Chapter

- Dairy free and delicious
- Excellent egg replacers
- Safe sweetening
- Oily considerations
- Gluten-free flours

Whether you've been gluten free and vegan for a while or you're just now dipping in your toe, you can be confident that there are healthful and conscious alternatives to everything. Replacing dairy and eggs in cooking and baking is easy and more affordable (both for your wallet and your body). Because our goal is to show you how delicious nutritious can be, in this chapter, we show you how to choose sweeteners that don't harm your waistline, your blood lab values, or even the flavor or textures of your desserts. Oil is a controversial ingredient that needs to be considered. We explain the facts about fat and its oil derivatives in this chapter, as well as provide general guidelines for substituting it in your diet.

Flour is one item you may have worried about once you determined your need to go gluten free. Worry no more! In the following pages, we guide you along in making healthy choices in the now-booming gluten-free market, enabling you to make any baked good you could ever desire. The chemistry behind baking is complex—especially when switching to gluten-free ingredients. This chapter gives you some tools you can use to transform your kitchen into a world of opportunity.

Ditching the Dairy

Do you really require dairy to be healthy and thrive? The correct answer is a resounding "no." In fact, it's quite the opposite. Humans are the only species to both continue drinking milk after weaning and to drink milk from other animals. We also happen to be the only species experiencing epidemic levels of chronic disease and obesity.

A vast majority of the world's population—approximately 70 percent—is intolerant to milk's sugar, lactose. Your production of lactase, the enzyme responsible for digesting lactose, naturally starts diminishing after age 2, which, coincidentally, is the appropriate time to begin weaning. Yet you're advised to continue consuming animal-based milk for life to promote adequate intake of calcium and other nutrients. Meanwhile, the incidences of intolerance or discomfort continue to grow. Maybe it's time to listen to the signals of our bodies and not force-feed them something they're not capable of digesting.

Believe it or not, dairy is also physiologically addicting. Casein, the primary protein in milk, causes the production of casomorphins in your body. These opiate-like compounds activate a hefty release of feel-good hormones, causing you to crave more. The solution? Cut out dairy, and after a few short weeks, your cravings will disappear.

And do we have some substitutions for you! Delicious plant-based milks, cheeses, sour cream, and other products step in to replace the dairy-based versions you've grown accustomed to.

Milk Madness

Have you checked out the wall of plant-based milks at your local grocery store lately? There used to be just soy milk and rice milk to choose from. Nowadays, you can find hemp milk, oat milk, almond milk, coconut milk, rice milk, 10 varieties of soy milk, and more. Flavors and brands vary widely. The hardest part is deciding among sweetened, unsweetened, vanilla, chocolate, plain, horchata, special holiday flavors, and whether you're going to go with a refrigerated or shelf-stable option!

Nutritionally speaking, opt for an unsweetened variety of any flavor. Hemp, oat, almond, and soy milks are the most nutrient-dense. Coconut milk is high in saturated fat, so we recommend limiting its use.

In culinary terms, soy milk is excellent for adding some creaminess, and hemp milk provides some grit and earthiness to your dishes. Rice milk is thinner and mild-flavored, while oat milk is thick, hearty, and mildly granular. Depending on the dish you're making, you can experiment with the diverse textures and flavors of all the beverages available.

DIY Nondairy Products

To save money and have full control over what goes into your products, you can make them yourself at home with few ingredients.

In Chapter 4, we give you a recipe for Awesome Almond Milk. Another way to make a nut or seed milk is to add 1 tablespoon nut or seed butter (try cashew, almond, or peanut butter) to 3 cups water and blend for 10 seconds.

Make your own vegan buttermilk by combining 1 tablespoon of an acid like lemon juice or vinegar, such as apple cider or white, with 1 cup unflavored, unsweetened soy milk or other nondairy milk. Allow it to sit for a few minutes to enable curdling to occur, and use it in our Bettermilk Biscuits recipe in Chapter 5. You can adjust the thickness by increasing or decreasing the amount of acid accordingly.

Chapter 6 is filled with all types of tantalizing plant-based cheeses, including sprinkles, sauces, spreads, and blocks. And in Chapter 9, we give you a recipe for homemade Tofu Sour Cream.

Easy Eggless Alternatives

Nutritionally, eggs are commonly considered a superior food. On the contrary, eggs are not the superstars they're cracked up to be. The yolks are high in cholesterol and fat (much of it saturated), and the whites are a concentrated source of animal protein.

Many people who contemplate veganism hesitate going all the way due to their concern of being able to cook and, especially, bake without eggs. Yet again, we have egg-cellent news about egg-free cooking and baking. Super substitutions exist to facilitate fluffy cakes, moist cookies, meatless loafs that bind, savory scrambles, and even soufflés that rise.

Because eggs play several culinary roles from binding to leavening and savory to sweet, what you use as a replacement is specific to the dish. You can pick up some commercial products or do it yourself with simple ingredients you probably have stocked in your kitchen already.

Commercial egg replacers are available online and possibly also in your local natural foods store. However, be wary of gluten in these products. Ener-G Egg Replacer and Orgran No Egg are gluten-free egg substitutes.

To replace 1 egg, most product packages recommend mixing 1½ teaspoons egg replacer with 2 tablespoons warm water. However, in some recipes, you may have better results by doubling the amount to 1 tablespoon egg replacer and 4 tablespoons water. Be sure to thoroughly and vigorously whisk the egg replacer and water together to fully dissolve it and to attain the desired consistency and proper functioning properties.

You can also easily replace eggs with whole foods to save cash and up the health ante. Remember that every recipe is special, and it's impossible to generalize perfectly. However, to start, let's look at some guidelines on how to substitute 1 egg in a recipe.

For binding in baked goods, use 2 tablespoons arrowroot or cornstarch, or 1 *flax egg*.

DEFINITION

Flax eggs are a phenomenal answer to egg-free cooking and baking. They look, taste, act, and feel like egg whites, yet they're healthy (hello, omega-3 fatty acids!), much less expensive, and work just as well. For an equivalent of 1 egg, combine 1 tablespoon ground flaxseeds or flaxseed meal with 3 tablespoons water, blend or whisk, and allow to sit for 5 minutes before using.

For added thickening and leavening properties, try ¼ cup unsweetened vegan yogurt or ¼ cup blended silken tofu. Depending on the recipe, you may need to add an additional ½ teaspoon baking powder or other leavening agent.

To add moisture in baked goods, use ¼ cup puréed fruit or vegetable such as applesauce, banana, zucchini, pumpkin, sweet potato, etc. Depending on the recipe, you may need to add an additional ½ teaspoon baking powder or other leavening agent.

For binding in a savory dish (like a casserole or loaf), substitute with ¼ cup blended silken tofu; 2 tablespoons vegetable purée, tahini, nut butter, or tomato paste; 1 flax egg; or 2 tablespoons cornstarch or arrowroot mixed with 2 tablespoons water.

Sugary Sweet

Sugar sneaks up on you under many different guises. Bold in cereals, baked goods, and candy, sugar also hides in items like pasta sauce, canned soup, "health" beverages, plant-based milks, barbecue sauce, and nutrition bars. But why does it matter?

Refined sweeteners like brown sugar, unbleached cane sugar or evaporated cane juice, high-fructose corn syrup, and even agave can wreak havoc on your health. They promote an acidic environment within the body that contributes to disease. Conditions associated with the consumption of sugar include tooth decay, diabetes, increased weight, obesity, premature aging, cancer, metabolic syndrome, depression, and anxiety. Regular consumption can also encourage the loss of important minerals like calcium, suppress immune function, and disturb brain chemistry. Worse, sugar is extraordinarily addicting. We suggest moderating your sweetener consumption if you feel that you aren't quite ready for eliminating it completely.

CORNUCOPIA

Many refined sweeteners aren't vegan, like honey, which comes from bees. Although they don't actually contain animal ingredients, many brands of white sugar are filtered using animal bone char to make them bright white, which is why we recommend only using unbleached cane sugar, turbinado sugar, and varieties of light or dark brown sugar.

Agave Nectar: Health or Hype?

Agave nectar has been touted as a health food in recent years and is often used as a vegan replacement for honey. However, it may not be all it's hyped up to be. In fact, it may even be harmful if used consistently.

Agave nectar has a low glycemic index value due to its high fructose content and has been marketed as such toward diabetics and those trying to lose weight. Ironically, its high fructose content is what negates any possible benefits for diabetics.

Fructose is a simple sugar that acts profoundly different in your body when compared to glucose because it's metabolized in the liver first instead of directly hitting the bloodstream. It turns into fat easier, increases blood triglyceride and insulin levels, induces insulin resistance, and is associated with elevated blood pressure and blood cholesterol.

Sucrose (table sugar) is about half fructose and half glucose. High-fructose corn syrup—commonly vilified and blamed as the source of chronic disease today—has approximately 55 percent fructose. Yet agave nectar gets between 70 and 90 percent of its sugar content from fructose, which makes some health-care professionals question its safety.

You may be wondering about fructose found in fruit. First of all, fruit contains lower levels of fructose. Also, because fruit is whole and includes fiber, vitamins, minerals, phytonutrients, and antioxidants, the fructose is absorbed much slower. Mother Nature has perfected the nutrient balance in her ready-to-eat products. We only get into trouble when we start manipulating them.

Whole-Food Sweeteners

Fortunately, when you go back to nature, you can find sweetness in its original packaging alongside fiber, vitamins, minerals, phytonutrients, and antioxidants. Fruit, dried fruit, dried fruit paste and syrup, maple syrup, and blackstrap molasses are excellent cooking and baking companions, and they add nutrition while they sweeten.

In Chapter 8, you'll find easy recipes to turn dried fruits like dates, raisins, prunes, and apricots into a paste that can replace honey, sugar, and other sweeteners in baked goods, dressings, sauces, and more. In some recipes, you can simply replace equal amounts of liquid sweetener with a fruit paste or maple syrup without significantly affecting the consistency of your final product.

Brown rice syrup is another liquid sweetener that's vegan and slightly superior nutritionally to table sugar, thanks to some potassium and more complex sugars. Be sure the package says "gluten free." Produced by fermenting brown rice with enzymes, the source of the enzymes determines whether or not the product is gluten free. If the enzymes are from barley, it's not gluten free. Some companies, including Lundberg Farms, use fungal enzymes instead, making their brown rice syrup gluten free.

Oil Slick

Fat is an important macronutrient required in your daily diet. However, to minimize your risk of disease and maintain your ideal body weight, your fat intake needs to stay on the lower side. Further, research points to a powerful difference in your body's response to the sources of fat you consume.

When eaten in its original form—from whole-plant sources like nuts, seeds, avocados, olives, and even leafy green vegetables—your body will respond positively to fat. All the adverse effects of fat discussed in the media and scientific literature are linked to the excess consumption of vegetable oils and animal products.

Not a Health Food

Oil is a processed food, a concentrated extraction comprised of 100 percent fat that provides approximately 120 calories per tablespoon. The fiber, vitamins, and minerals have been removed. Several renowned physicians, including Drs. John McDougall, Dean Ornish, and Caldwell Esselstyn, have had dramatic results reversing heart disease on a low-fat, oil-free diet. They literally took patients who were told by their doctors they had irreversible heart damage and were nearing death and helped them fully recover.

Health-promoting foods are nutrient dense, providing maximum nutrition with the least calories. Oil is the opposite. Compare 1 tablespoon flaxseed oil, which has 120 calories, 14 grams fat, 0 fiber, and no vitamins and minerals (save for a touch of vitamin E) to 1 tablespoon whole flaxseeds, which has 36 calories, 2 grams fiber, 1.7 grams protein, and 3 grams fat. The flaxseeds also contain some B vitamins, vitamin E, calcium, magnesium, potassium, phosphorus, and iron.

Similarly, 1 cup olives provides 155 calories; 1 gram protein; 8 grams carbohydrates; 4 grams fiber; 14 grams fat; vitamins A, C, E, and K; calcium; iron; magnesium; phosphorus; potassium; selenium; and sodium. Compare that to 1 cup extra-virgin olive oil, which contains 2,016 calories; 0 carbs, protein, or fiber; 224 grams fat; 28 milligrams vitamin E (the RDA is 15 mg for an adult); and no minerals.

Two popular oils misguidedly publicized for their health benefits are coconut and fish oil. Coconut oil has 87 percent of its total fat and calories consisting of saturated fat. This type of fat contributes greatly to elevated cholesterol levels. Fish oil is a cocktail of contaminants. Fish are jam-packed with toxins, including mercury, PCBs, dioxin, and DDT. Once concentrated into an oil, the level of these harmful compounds increases exponentially. Other potential adverse effects of fish oil supplementation include increased risk of bleeding, prevention of blood clotting, decreased blood pressure, and increased blood sugar.

If you opt to use oils on occasion, we suggest selecting expeller- or cold-pressed oils to enhance flavor and color quality. These are less processed than their standard counterparts, which are refined, bleached, and deodorized using harsh chemicals like hexane. For a raw or cold-prepared dish, like a salad, cold-pressed oils (like hemp or flax) would be the best choice because they cannot be heated above 90 degrees due to their low smoke point. For cooked dishes, expeller-pressed oils (like olive or peanut) can withstand higher temperatures and are superior for sautéeing, stovetop cooking, and oven baking.

When using margarine, it's crucial to avoid nonhydrogenated options and the harmful effects of trans fatty acids.

Oil-Free Cooking and Baking

The beauty of reducing the oil in your diet is that you may not even miss it. Cooking and baking can be easily modified to produce quality, luscious cuisine. Oil-free stovetop cooking is extremely simple. Essentially, all you need to do is replace the oil with water, vegetable broth, juice, (flavored) vinegar, wine, or beer. Often you'll need to use a greater amount of one of these liquids to replace the particular oil called for in the recipe. So closely monitor the ingredients in your pan to avoid burning them, and keep in mind that you can easily add a bit more to the pan to help prevent foods from sticking.

In sauces and dressings, oil provides flavor, creaminess, and moisture. Flavor can also be enhanced with herbs, spices, vinegars, and extracts, which can help you to use minimal amounts of oil—or in some instances, none at all—without significantly altering the flavor of the final product. You may not even notice a difference. To substitute the creaminess of oil, try incorporating hemp seeds, flaxseeds, white cannellini beans, silken tofu, or our Oil Replacer in Chapter 9 instead. In terms of moisture, several options are available, depending on the nature of what you're whipping up. All the aforementioned stovetop cooking liquid options would also work for certain sauces and dressings. Other alternatives include plant-based milks, freshly juiced vegetables or fruits, unsweetened coconut water, tomato juice or sauce, and brewed tea.

With baking, oil or margarine have two major roles: prevent sticking and provide moisture. Using parchment paper, a *Silpat liner*, or silicone bakeware helps alleviate the first issue. For moisture, you can substitute the amount of oil or margarine in a recipe with up to half the amount of mashed bananas, applesauce, puréed prunes, silken tofu, or mashed avocado. Because using one of these substitutes may slightly alter the final flavor of the baked item, try to base your substitution selection around what will best complement the other ingredients in the recipe. Using one of these tasty options not only helps enhance the texture and flavor of baked goods, but also helps cut the fat content of the final product.

DEFINITION

Silpat liners are reusable, nonstick baking mats made of fiberglass and silicone often used to line cookie sheets and baking pans as an alternative to lightly oiling or using parchment paper. They can turn any work surface or counter into a nonstick surface, so bakers often use them for rolling out pastry or cookie dough, kneading and shaping breads and other baked goods, or when making candy. Silpat liners can be used at temperatures varying from 40°F to 482°F.

Flour Power

There's much confusion when it comes to flour and nutrition. The majority of commercial products, recipes, and ingredients out there use heavily processed, refined flours. Fortunately for anyone with gluten-intolerance, wheat is the primary grain used for making those flours. Think of it as a blessing in disguise. You are forced into choosing healthier whole-grain, legume, nut, and seed-based flours instead.

Homemade Flours

Companies such as Bob's Red Mill and Arrowhead Mills produce gluten-free flour products made from a wide assortment of grains, nuts, and legumes, including brown rice, almond, chickpea/garbanzo bean, fava bean, black bean, quinoa, corn, and oats. They also make preformulated packaged blends for general baking, pancakes and waffles, pizza crust, and more. Think of the possibilities!

These gluten-free, alternative flour blends and baking mixes can often be used measure for measure as a replacement for unbleached all-purpose flour and whole-wheat pastry flour in your gluten-free vegan baking. You can find them in most grocery and natural foods stores as well as online.

One of the products you can use for the baked recipes in this book is Bob's Red Mill Gluten-Free All-Purpose Baking Flour. It consists of chickpea/garbanzo bean flour, potato starch, tapioca flour, sorghum flour, and fava flour. However, in some recipes, we prefer our homemade gluten-free baking blend we call Beverly's Baking Blend.

Beverly's Baking Blend

This blend is based on a commonly used ratio of gluten-free flours and starches, but it uses a bit more brown rice flour and seems to work extremely well in many of our baked goods.

Yield:	Prep time:
8 cups	2 or 3 minutes

5½ cups brown rice flour

1½ cups potato starch

1 cup tapioca starch

1. In a large bowl, whisk together brown rice flour, potato starch, and tapioca starch.

2. Transfer to an airtight container or zipper-lock bag for up to 3 months at room temperature, or 6 months in the refrigerator.

Variation: Try replacing 2 cups brown rice flour with an equal amount of almond meal, chickpea/garbanzo bean flour, or garfava bean flour.

> **CORNUCOPIA**
>
> Be sure to measure your gluten-free flours and starches by spooning them into a measuring cup and then leveling it off with the back of a knife or spoon. Dipping or scooping them into your measuring cup could ultimately result in too much or too little of the amount called for in the recipe.

Component Chemistry

Baking is a chemistry experiment. To achieve the perfect density, texture, rise, color, and flavor, the ingredients need to be in just the right combination. Every item plays an important role. When you omit gluten—an important protein in baking—you need to compensate with accurate quantities of other proteins. Substitutions and replacements require precision and a sharp eye. Let's take a look at some ingredients that act as stars and co-stars in gluten-free baking.

Agar-agar is a gelatin-like substance derived from red algae. Sold in both flake and powder form, agar-agar can be used as a thickening and stabilizing agent in cooking and baking. Because of its similarity to gelatin, it can be used to make jellies, custards, puddings, and vegetarian aspics.

Prepare agar-agar as you would an animal-based gelatin, dissolving it in a liquid over heat, bringing it to a boil, simmering it until thickened, and allowing it to cool. Or you can use undissolved agar powder as an ingredient in recipes such as the Multi-Grain Sandwich Bread (recipe in Chapter 5). Extremely high in fiber, agar-agar is also used as a laxative.

Arrowroot is a perennial herb grown in rainforest habitats that yields an edible starch obtained from the roots. Naturally gluten free, arrowroot makes an excellent replacement for wheat flour in baking. As an effective thickener, arrowroot is more stable to temperature and acidity than other starches. It also maintains a clear color and adds a transparent sheen to pies, jams, and sauces. Arrowroot has a neutral taste.

When adding arrowroot to liquids, the mixture tends to become clumpy. To avoid this, mix an equal amount of cool liquid into the starch until it forms a paste. Then whisk the paste back into the liquid to thicken.

Baking powder is a dry ingredient used to increase volume and lighten or leaven baked goods. It works via an acid-base chemical reaction where carbon dioxide gas is released, causing bubbles to expand, thereby enabling the product to rise. The ingredients that make up baking powder include the alkaline substance baking soda (sodium bicarbonate), an acid like cream of tartar, and an inert starch to absorb the moisture.

The source of the starch usually comes from cornstarch, but it can vary and sometimes wheat starch is used. Therefore, it's critical to look for "gluten free" on the label. To avoid concern, you can easily make baking powder at home with the following simple recipe.

DIY Baking Powder

For an easy way to prevent gluten in your baking powder, try this simple combination.

Yield:	Prep time:
4 teaspoons	2 minutes

2 tsp. cream of tartar   1 tsp. cornstarch

1 tsp. baking soda

1. In a small bowl, mix cream of tartar, baking soda, and cornstarch together until well combined.

2. Use immediately or store in an airtight container for up to 6 months.

Cornstarch is one of the most commonly used starches in baking and food processing. Essentially, it's the refined starch of the endosperm of the corn kernel. Cornstarch functions as a gluten-free vegan thickener and is also often mixed with cold liquid to make into a paste before adding to a recipe to avoid clumps.

Guar gum is essentially the endosperm of guar beans ground into a fine powder. Guar gum is a soluble fiber that thickens tremendously when mixed with water. It has many applications in cooking and baking and is an economical choice because a little goes a long way. Guar gum contributes to viscosity, helps maintain stability, and acts as an emulsifier. When mixed with xanthan gum, they enhance viscosity. In baked goods, guar gum helps condition the dough and retain moisture.

Potato starch is another starch used as a thickener, especially in soups, gravies, stews, and sauces. It's also a gluten-free vegan way to add moistness in baking.

Rapid-rise active yeast is a variety of baker's yeast that's an instant version of active dry yeast. Active dry yeast is a living microorganism that acts as a leavening agent when making breads and other baked products. The live cells—which are enclosed by dry, dead cells—must be hydrated to activate. When moisture is added, the yeast ferments the sugars into carbon dioxide and ethanol, causing the rise to occur. The rapid-rise variety is made with smaller granules and a higher percentage of live microorganisms to expedite both the rate at which it dissolves in dough and at which it causes the dough to rise.

You can use rapid-rise active yeast when the recipe calls for active dry yeast, but you only need to allow the dough to rise once, not twice, as is commonly done with active yeast, making the rising time shorter. Note that the rise may be smaller in the finished product.

Salt is used in baked goods to enhance flavor, help strengthen the protein in the dough, and steady the fermentation rate. Because it provides functional support to baked goods, and works as part of the chemical reactions, it's necessary to include it in those recipes.

Sorghum, also known as milo, is a cereal grass cultivated to make flour or for use as a feed grain. Nutritionally dense with fiber, iron, phosphorus, potassium, calcium, and protein, sorghum adds volume, texture, crumb, and a slightly nutty flavor to baked goods.

Tapioca starch originates from the cassava root, a starchy tuber that resembles a potato. In dough, tapioca gelatinizes during baking and adds chewiness to the texture. This also enables the finished product to maintain structure.

Xanthan gum is similar to guar gum in its characteristics and uses. Made from a microorganism called *Xanthomonas campestris*, it is effective at thickening, stabilizing, and emulsifying dressings and sauces in tiny amounts. Similar to gluten in its function, xanthan gum helps provide the gumminess in dough when used in baking. It can be found packaged and in the bulk section of most grocery and natural foods stores as well as through online sources. Although xanthan gum is vegan, it may not necessarily be gluten free because it's sometimes produced using wheat. As always, be sure to read the package for the words "gluten free."

A Grain of Salt

To salt or not to salt seems to be a popular question. Several issues pop into play when it comes to the world's most popular seasoning.

Sodium is necessary in your diet to maintain fluid balance, regulate blood pressure and blood volume, and transmit nerve impulses. Under normal conditions and without sweating, your body only needs 180 milligrams per day. Even though the 2010 Dietary Guidelines and the Institute of Medicine's Food and Nutrition Board both recommend a maximum intake of 1,500 milligrams daily, the average person consumes closer to 3,500! Close to 80 percent of dietary sodium comes from processed and restaurant foods. A mere teaspoon of table salt contains more than 2,300 milligrams sodium.

Some Thoughts on Sodium

Excess sodium in the diet negatively impacts your health via several avenues. It notoriously raises blood pressure, which increases your risk for heart attacks and strokes. High sodium intake also promotes osteoporosis by enhancing calcium loss in the urine and stresses the kidneys, stomach, and blood vessels.

On the upside, iodized salt is an excellent vehicle for adequate consumption of iodine. You don't need much to get your daily allowance—only $\frac{3}{8}$ to $\frac{1}{2}$ teaspoon gives you the Dietary Reference Intakes (DRI) of 15 micrograms iodine, as long as the salt you use is iodized. Sea salts and other gourmet salts are not iodized but provide trace amounts of other minerals, usually below recommended levels.

Have you ever noticed that the more salt you use, the more you need to actually taste it? Like sugar, salt has an addictive component, and your taste buds adjust quickly to change in either direction, more or less. So use salt in moderation.

Subbing Salt

Many different foods are naturally (or not-so-naturally) high in sodium and can be used to add saltiness to your foods. Sun-dried tomatoes, wheat-free tamari, and sea vegetables are healthful ingredients you can use in your cooking.

Some excellent commercial salt substitutions, such as Dragunara's Slim Spice seasoning and Benson's Table Tasty, are also available. Kelp or dulse shakers, other sea veggie blends, and nutritional yeast are salt free but provide salty flavoring and are easy to find at a natural foods store or online.

Throughout this book, we share tricks and tips for substituting and creating magical gluten-free vegan dishes. Turn to the next chapter, try some recipes, and adapt the methods to expand your gluten-free vegan substitution repertoire.

The Least You Need to Know

- Dairy is easier than ever before to substitute, thanks to a variety of nut- and plant-based milks.
- Have no worries about replacing eggs in cooking and even baking with several plant-based egg alternatives.
- Refined sweeteners can wreak havoc on your health. Opt for whole-food options to sweeten your culinary creations.
- Most recipes can be created without or with limited amounts of oil without sacrificing the finished product.
- Flours made from other whole grains, nuts, legumes, and other ingredients can enhance your pantry and your inventory of food options.

Off to a Good Start

To help get you off to a good start on your gluten-free vegan diet, we begin to share our recipes that utilize these delicious, nutritious ingredients. And we can say that with authority, since one of us is a trained plant-based dietitian and the other is an experienced vegan chef and baker. We'll be by your side all the way, showing you how to create gluten-free meals you'll love.

Some of the ingredients in the following recipes will be things you're already using in your meal preparations. Others might be new and perhaps a bit confusing (or oddly or strangely named), but you'll be using them like an old pro in no time.

As it's important to start your day off right by having a nourishing breakfast, this is the focus of our first recipe chapter. In it, we share ideas for cold and quick options, as well as gluten-free vegan versions of classic diner and brunch specialties. If you're someone who often has to make a mad dash out the door and needs more portable on-the-go breakfast ideas, you'll be delighted by the grab-and-go biscuits, muffins, and sweet quick breads in Chapter 5. And because it can be difficult to find gluten-free vegan sliced breads, buns, pies, and pizza crusts in the corner grocery store, we included recipes for all these in Part 2.

We finish this "building a good solid foundation" part by providing recipes for making your own homemade dairy-free cheeses of varying flavors and textures.

Breakfast A-Go-Go

In This Chapter

- Energizing breakfast beverages
- Sensational skillet-cooked dishes
- Eggless scrambles and quiches

Maintaining a gluten-free vegan diet is super easy with these delicious and simple breakfast recipes. In this chapter, you find recipe ideas for fast and easy breakfasts, including one that requires no cooking at all, that are perfect for hectic Monday mornings or when you're short on time.

Revamps of classic breakfast items, with an effort to make them healthier yet flavorful, include options such as pancakes, waffles, and French toast. We also include a new and improved diner-style blue-plate special of scrambled eggs (really, tofu) and home fries. To further boost your comfort food indulgences, add selections like Smoky Tempeh Un-Bacon and Savory Sausages found in Chapter 12, and you're ready for breakfast.

Awesome Almond Milk

Almond milk is a tasty dairy-free milk alternative for the gluten-free vegan, and it's surprisingly easy to make at home. Enjoy as a beverage or use measure for measure in recipes.

Yield:	Prep time:	Serving size:
3 cups	5 minutes, plus 6 or more hours soak time	1 cup

1 cup raw almonds	4 cups water

1. In a small bowl, combine almonds and 1 cup water. Set aside to soak for 6 hours or overnight.

2. Drain off soaking water, rinse almonds, and drain again. Squeeze each almond between your thumb and forefinger to remove and discard skin.

3. In a blender, place almonds and remaining 3 cups water, and blend for 1 or 2 minutes or until smooth and creamy.

4. Strain through cheesecloth or a fine mesh sieve. Discard almond meal pulp, or save it for later use. Store in an airtight container in the refrigerator for 3 or 4 days.

Variation: You can also use this method to make other nut- or seed-based milks by replacing the almonds with cashews, hazelnuts, Brazil nuts, or hemp or sunflower seeds. Or for **Sweet Vanilla Almond Milk,** add 2 or 3 pitted dried dates and a small amount of alcohol-free vanilla extract or *raw vanilla bean powder*.

> **DEFINITION**
>
> **Raw vanilla bean powder** is made by grinding dried, whole vanilla beans. It has a very intense flavor; a ½ teaspoon vanilla bean powder is the equivalent of 1 teaspoon vanilla extract. You can find raw vanilla bean powder in natural foods stores and through online sources such as mountainroseherbs.com.

Tropical Greens Delight

Take a trip to the tropics with the island-reminiscent flavors of coconut, mango, and lime. This brightly colored, frosty delight will cool you down and offer a little kick of spice.

Yield:	Prep time:	Serving size:
2½ cups	5 minutes	1¼ cups

1 cup frozen mango chunks	1 cup baby spinach, tightly packed
1 cup frozen pineapple chunks	¼ cup lime juice
1½ cups unsweetened *coconut water*	¼ tsp. cayenne

1. In a blender, place mango chunks, pineapple chunks, coconut water, baby spinach, lime juice, and cayenne, and blend for 30 to 60 seconds or until smooth and creamy.

2. Evenly divide mixture between 2 glasses, and serve immediately.

Variation: If you prefer a less-spicy version, you can reduce or omit the cayenne. You can also replace the mango chunks with papaya. If you can't find frozen fruit, use the same amount of fresh fruit and add 1 cup ice cubes.

> **DEFINITION**
>
> **Coconut water** is the clear to translucent liquid found inside a young, green coconut. It's mild and sweet in flavor and rich in electrolytes, making it the perfect natural sports drink. Find it in grocery and natural foods stores and wholesale shopping centers.

Fantastic French Toast

By combining a few pantry staples with our Sweet Vanilla Almond Milk, you can transform humble slices of bread into a fantastic and filling breakfast within minutes.

Yield:	Prep time:	Cook time:	Serving size:
8 slices	5 to 7 minutes	8 to 10 minutes	2 slices

1½ cups Sweet Vanilla Almond Milk (variation earlier in this chapter), soy milk, or other nondairy milk

3 TB. chickpea/garbanzo bean flour

1½ TB. cornstarch or arrowroot

1½ TB. nutritional yeast flakes

1 TB. maple syrup or sorghum syrup

2 tsp. alcohol-free vanilla extract or 1 tsp. raw vanilla bean powder

1 tsp. ground cinnamon

8 slices Multi-Grain Sandwich Bread (recipe in Chapter 5), Banana-Date Bread (recipe in Chapter 5), or other gluten-free bread

1. In a large, shallow casserole dish or pie pan, combine Sweet Vanilla Almond Milk, chickpea/garbanzo bean flour, cornstarch, nutritional yeast flakes, maple syrup, vanilla extract, and cinnamon, and whisk well.

2. Place 4 Multi-Grain Sandwich Bread slices into almond milk mixture, flip slices over to coat other side, and leave to soak for 2 minutes.

3. Lightly oil a large, nonstick skillet, and place over medium heat. (Or use a griddle.)

4. Using a fork, carefully remove bread slices from Vanilla Almond Milk mixture, and place them into the hot skillet.

5. Cook bread slices for 1 or 2 minutes or until golden brown on the bottom. Flip over bread with a spatula, and cook for 1 or 2 more minutes or until golden brown on the other side.

6. While first batch cooks, repeat soaking procedure for remaining 4 slices of bread. Lightly oil the skillet again, and repeat procedure for remaining bread slices. Serve hot with maple syrup, sorghum syrup, or other toppings of choice.

Variation: For added flavor, add 1 teaspoon finely grated orange zest and ¼ teaspoon freshly grated nutmeg to the Sweet Vanilla Almond Milk mixture.

MEATLESS AND WHEATLESS

You can cook up large batches of French toast, pancakes, or waffles; place them in an airtight container or zipper-lock bag; and freeze them for later use. Then, simply remove servings as desired from the freezer and reheat for a few minutes in a 350°F oven, a dry skillet, a toaster, or in the microwave. Quick and easy breakfast!

Buckwheat-Flax Pancakes

These pancakes are rich in fiber and protein, with a slightly nutty flavor and color, thanks to combining buckwheat and brown rice flours with ground flaxseeds.

Yield:	Prep time:	Cook time:	Serving size:
8 pancakes	8 to 10 minutes	15 to 20 minutes	1 pancake

6 TB. water

2 TB. ground flaxseeds or flaxseed meal

1 cup *buckwheat flour*

1 cup brown rice flour

1 TB. aluminum-free baking powder

1½ tsp. ground cinnamon

Pinch sea salt

2½ cups soy milk or other nondairy milk

1½ TB. maple syrup, gluten-free brown rice syrup, or sorghum syrup

1 TB. sunflower oil

1. In a medium bowl, combine water and flaxseeds, and let sit for 5 minutes.

2. In a large bowl, combine buckwheat flour, brown rice flour, baking powder, cinnamon, and sea salt, and whisk well.

3. Whisk soy milk, maple syrup, and sunflower oil into flaxseed mixture. Add wet ingredients to dry ingredients, and whisk well to combine.

4. Lightly oil a medium or large nonstick skillet, and place over medium heat. (Or use a griddle.)

5. Pour ½ cup batter per pancake into the hot skillet.

6. Cook for 2 or 3 minutes or until edges of pancake are slightly dry and bubbles appear on top. Flip over pancake with a spatula, and cook for 2 or 3 more minutes or until golden brown on the other side. As needed, lightly oil the skillet again and repeat procedure for remaining batter. Serve hot with maple syrup, sorghum syrup, or other toppings of choice.

Variation: Feel free to add sliced bananas, chopped nuts, or seeds to the portioned pancake batter prior to flipping. For **Gingerbread Pancakes,** add an additional 1 teaspoon ground cinnamon, along with 1½ teaspoons ground ginger, ½ teaspoon ground cloves or allspice, and ½ teaspoon freshly ground nutmeg.

Plant-Based Dietitian Recommends: Omit oil. To prevent sticking, be sure to use a safe nonstick skillet or griddle, as discussed in Chapter 2.

DEFINITION

Buckwheat flour is made by finely grinding buckwheat groats. Although it has "wheat" in its name, buckwheat is not related to wheat at all. It's neither a grain nor a grass, but rather a fruit seed, a member of the rhubarb family. It's gluten free and is a good plant source of protein because it contains all eight essential amino acids.

Sorghum-Corn Cakes with Berries

Although cornmeal is a key ingredient in these pancakes, sorghum flour and syrup are really what give them a slightly sweet and unique flavor.

Yield:	Prep time:	Cook time:	Serving size:
8 pancakes	5 to 7 minutes	15 to 20 minutes	1 pancake

1 cup medium-grind yellow cornmeal

$\frac{1}{3}$ cup sorghum flour

3 TB. chickpea/garbanzo bean flour

1 TB. aluminum-free baking powder

$\frac{1}{4}$ tsp. sea salt

1 cup soy milk or other nondairy milk

$\frac{1}{2}$ cup water

1 TB. *sorghum syrup,* gluten-free brown rice syrup, or maple syrup

$\frac{1}{2}$ tsp. alcohol-free vanilla extract

1 (10-oz.) pkg. frozen blueberries or mixed berries, unthawed, or $1\frac{1}{2}$ cups fresh berries

1. In a medium bowl, combine cornmeal, sorghum flour, chickpea/garbanzo bean flour, baking powder, and sea salt, and whisk well. Add soy milk, water, sorghum syrup, and vanilla extract, and whisk well to combine. Gently fold in blueberries.

2. Lightly oil a medium or large nonstick skillet, and place over medium heat. (Or use a griddle.)

3. Pour $\frac{1}{2}$ cup batter per pancake into the hot skillet.

4. Cook for 2 or 3 minutes or until edges of pancake are slightly dry and bubbles appear on top. Flip over pancake with a spatula and cook for 2 or 3 more minutes or until golden brown on the other side. As needed, lightly oil the skillet again and repeat procedure for remaining batter. Serve hot with sorghum syrup, maple syrup, or other toppings of choice.

Variation: Feel free to replace the blueberries with other fresh or frozen fruit as desired. For **Savory Sorghum Cakes,** omit the blueberries and vanilla extract, and instead add 1 cup frozen or fresh cut corn kernels, $\frac{1}{2}$ cup diced red bell pepper, and $\frac{1}{4}$ cup thinly sliced green onions, and serve topped with salsa or sorghum syrup.

Plant-Based Dietitian Recommends: To prevent sticking, be sure to use a safe nonstick skillet or griddle instead of oil.

DEFINITION

Sorghum syrup, also referred to as sorghum molasses, is made from the sweet sorghum variety of the cereal grain sorghum. In a process similar to making molasses from sugarcane, the sweet juices that have been extracted from the plants' stalks are boiled down to create mild-flavored, amber-colored syrup. Use sorghum syrup as a table syrup on top of hot cereals, pancakes, or biscuits, as well as to flavor beans, barbecue sauce, breads, cakes, and other baked goods.

Orange and Vanilla–Kissed Waffles

These crisp waffles, flavored with fresh orange zest and juice, cinnamon, and a generous amount of vanilla extract, are guaranteed to get you rave reviews.

Yield:	Prep time:	Cook time:	Serving size:
6 waffles	7 to 10 minutes	15 to 20 minutes	1 waffle

1⅓ cups soy milk or other nondairy milk

⅔ cup orange juice

½ cup applesauce

1½ TB. gluten-free brown rice syrup or maple syrup

1 TB. alcohol-free vanilla extract or 1½ tsp. raw vanilla bean powder

1⅓ cups brown rice flour

⅔ cup chickpea/garbanzo bean flour

6 TB. tapioca starch

1½ tsp. aluminum-free baking powder

1 tsp. ground cinnamon

1 tsp. orange zest

½ tsp. baking soda

¼ tsp. sea salt

1. In a medium bowl, combine soy milk and orange juice, and let sit for 5 minutes. Add applesauce, brown rice syrup, and vanilla extract, and stir well to combine.

2. In a large bowl, combine brown rice flour, chickpea/garbanzo bean flour, tapioca starch, baking powder, cinnamon, orange zest, baking soda, and sea salt, and whisk well. Add wet ingredients to dry ingredients, and whisk well to combine.

3. Lightly oil a waffle iron and preheat according to the manufacturer's instructions.

4. Depending on the size of your waffle iron, ladle ⅔ to ¾ cup batter onto the iron and cook according to manufacturer's instructions or until golden brown. Repeat procedure for remaining batter. Serve hot with maple syrup, jam, or other toppings of choice.

Variation: For a more traditional flavor, or as we like to call them, **Home-Style Waffles,** omit the orange zest and juice, and replace with 2½ tablespoons lemon juice, and use 1¾ cups soy milk instead of 1⅓ cups.

Plant-Based Dietitian Recommends: To prevent sticking, be sure to use a safe nonstick waffle iron instead of oil.

MEATLESS AND WHEATLESS

If the recipe you're preparing calls for both the zest and juice of a citrus fruit, like in this recipe, first remove the zest either with a zester or grater. Then, cut the citrus fruit in half, and squeeze or ream each half as desired.

Go Green Tofu Scramble

To further boost the nutritional benefits of this protein-packed scramble, the curry-flavored tofu and green veggies are sautéed in vegetable broth rather than oil.

Yield:	Prep time:	Cook time:	Serving size:
4 cups	10 minutes	8 to 10 minutes	²/₃ cup

1 lb. firm, extra-firm, or *super firm tofu*

4 to 6 TB. low-sodium vegetable broth

1¹/₂ TB. nutritional yeast flakes

1 TB. wheat-free tamari

¹/₄ tsp. curry powder or turmeric

¹/₄ tsp. smoked paprika or sweet paprika

¹/₄ tsp. freshly ground black pepper

4 cups lacinato (Italian) kale, green kale, or baby spinach, stems removed, and roughly chopped

²/₃ cup green bell pepper, diced

¹/₃ cup green onion, thinly sliced

2 TB. garlic, minced

¹/₄ cup chopped fresh cilantro

1. Place a large, nonstick skillet over medium heat. Using your fingers, crumble tofu into the skillet. Add 3 tablespoons vegetable broth, nutritional yeast flakes, tamari, curry powder, smoked paprika, and pepper, and stir well with a spatula. Cook, stirring often, for 2 minutes.

2. Add kale, green bell pepper, and 1 to 3 more tablespoons vegetable broth, as needed to prevent sticking, and continue to cook, stirring often, for 2 more minutes.

3. Add green onion and garlic, and continue to cook, stirring often, for 2 or 3 more minutes or until desired doneness. Stir in cilantro, remove from heat, and serve. Depending on the type of tofu used, your scramble will have a slightly soft to very firm texture after cooking.

Variation: You can also use the scramble as a filling for breakfast burritos. For a **Southwestern-Style Scramble,** use turmeric instead of curry powder, add ¹/₂ teaspoon chili powder to season the tofu, replace the kale with ¹/₂ cup cooked black beans and ²/₃ cup diced red bell pepper, and top individual servings with salsa as desired.

Mediterranean Eggless Quiche

Having friends or family over for brunch and not sure what to make? This savory quiche is made with blended tofu and a generous assortment of vegetables and topped with tangy kalamata olives and slices of juicy tomato.

Yield:	Prep time:	Cook time:	Serving size:
1 (9-inch) quiche	15 to 20 minutes	40 to 50 minutes	1 piece

1 batch of pastry for Gluten-Free Piecrust (recipe in Chapter 5)

1 lb. firm or extra-firm tofu, crumbled

$\frac{1}{2}$ cup soy milk or other nondairy milk

2 TB. arrowroot

2 TB. nutritional yeast flakes

$\frac{1}{2}$ tsp. agar powder or $1\frac{1}{2}$ tsp. agar-agar flakes

1 tsp. Dijon mustard

$\frac{1}{2}$ tsp. sea salt

$\frac{1}{4}$ tsp. turmeric

$\frac{1}{4}$ tsp. smoked paprika or sweet paprika

$\frac{1}{8}$ tsp. freshly ground black pepper or garlic pepper

$\frac{1}{4}$ cup chopped fresh basil or parsley (preferably Italian flat-leaf parsley)

$\frac{1}{2}$ cup zucchini, cut into quarters lengthwise and thinly sliced

1 TB. low-sodium vegetable broth or water

$\frac{1}{2}$ cup artichoke hearts, roughly chopped

1 TB. garlic, minced

$\frac{1}{4}$ tsp. crushed red pepper flakes

3 cups baby spinach, roughly chopped

3 TB. kalamata olives or other olives of choice, pitted and cut lengthwise into strips

1 large Roma tomato, thinly sliced

1. Preheat the oven to 375°F.

2. Prepare pastry for Gluten-Free Piecrust according to the recipe instructions, and shape into a disc. Chill pastry dough disc for 30 minutes.

3. For easier rolling, place chilled pastry dough disc between 2 (12×16-inch) pieces of parchment paper, and roll into a 12-inch circle. Remove and discard the top sheet of parchment paper. Flip pastry dough into pie pan, and remove and discard remaining parchment paper. Trim overhanging edge of pastry dough about 1 inch from the outer edge of the pie pan. Gently press down on outer edge to seal and flute edges as desired.

4. In a blender or food processor fitted with an S blade, place tofu, soy milk, arrowroot, nutritional yeast flakes, agar powder, Dijon mustard, sea salt, turmeric, smoked paprika, and pepper, and process for 1 or 2 minutes or until smooth. Scrape down sides of the container with a spatula, add basil, and process for 15 more seconds.

5. Place a medium, nonstick skillet over medium heat. Add zucchini and vegetable broth, and cook, stirring often, for 1 minute. Add artichoke hearts, garlic, and crushed red pepper flakes, and cook, stirring often, for 1 minute. Add spinach and cook, stirring often, for 1 more minute or until just wilted. Remove from heat.

6. Pour half of tofu mixture into prepared piecrust, top with cooked vegetable mixture, and top with remaining tofu mixture. Using a spatula or spoon, gently swirl two mixtures together and then smooth top.

7. Scatter kalamata olives over tofu mixture, and arrange Roma tomato slices in a circular pattern over top. Bake for 35 to 45 minutes or until filling is firm to the touch and dry on top. Remove from the oven. Allow quiche to cool for 15 minutes before cutting. Serve warm, cold, or at room temperature as desired.

Variation: Feel free to replace the recommended vegetables with an equal amount of other vegetables such as mushrooms, bell peppers, and broccoli, and sauté them in a similar manner as described in the recipe.

MEATLESS AND WHEATLESS

If you're intimidated by making your own piecrust or simply not in the mood for one, you can still make this quiche. Simply assemble the remaining quiche ingredients in a similar manner in a lightly oiled 9-inch pie pan, and bake for 30 to 40 minutes.

Oven-Roasted Home Fries

These colorful, oven-baked home fries are prepared with earthy potatoes, rutabagas, sweet potatoes, juicy bell peppers, and red onion, with a fraction of the oil typically used when skillet frying.

Yield:	Prep time:	Cook time:	Serving size:
4½ cups	5 to 7 minutes	35 to 40 minutes	¾ cup

2 cups red-skinned potatoes, cut into 1-in. cubes

2 cups rutabaga, peeled and cut into 1-in. cubes

2 cups sweet potatoes, cut into 1-in. cubes

1½ TB. low-sodium vegetable broth

1½ TB. olive or other oil

¾ tsp. dried basil

¾ tsp. dried thyme

¾ tsp. garlic granules or garlic powder

½ tsp. smoked paprika or chili powder

¼ tsp. sea salt

¼ tsp. freshly ground black pepper or garlic pepper

⅔ cup red onion, diced

⅔ cup green bell pepper, diced

⅔ cup red bell pepper, diced

1. Preheat the oven to 425°F. Line a cookie sheet with parchment paper or a Silpat liner.

2. In a large bowl, combine potatoes, rutabaga, sweet potatoes, vegetable broth, olive oil, basil, thyme, garlic granules, smoked paprika, sea salt, and pepper. Using your hands, toss mixture until evenly coated.

3. Transfer mixture to the prepared cookie sheet, and spread out to form a single layer. Bake for 20 minutes.

4. Remove from the oven, stir with a spatula, and spread out into a single layer. Scatter red onion, green bell pepper, and red bell pepper over top, and bake for 15 to 20 more minutes or until desired doneness. Remove from the oven, and serve hot.

Variation: If you don't like the flavor of rutabaga or sweet potatoes, feel free to replace them with blue or purple potatoes, or just use additional red-skinned potatoes. You can also replace the dried basil and thyme with 1½ teaspoons herbes de Provence.

Plant-Based Dietitian Recommends: Substitute 3 tablespoons additional vegetable broth for the olive oil, for a total of 4½ tablespoons vegetable broth.

AGAINST THE GRAIN

Prolonged exposure to light during storage can cause raw potatoes to turn green, which is why farmers recommend storing them in a cool, dark, well-ventilated place. Green potatoes may contain a substance called solanine, which can be toxic as well as give them a bitter flavor. However, you don't need to discard the whole potato if only part of it is green or sprouted. Just remove these imperfections and proceed with your preparations from there.

Bountiful Breads and Baked Goods

In This Chapter

- Sweet and savory muffins and quick breads
- Yeasted bread and buns
- Pie and pizza crusts

Baking with gluten-free flours is a challenge because wheat is such a widely used ingredient that's included in most recipes. This is why so many gluten-free bakers rely on eggs, butter, and dairy products to lighten and bind their baked goods and breads. Gluten-free vegan recipe development is a bit trickier. We introduced you to some general guidelines in Chapter 3 for egg and dairy substitutions. In this chapter, you learn how to implement them for delicious and effective results.

Don't be afraid to experiment with certain ingredients in your baking. For instance, instead of just water, use some unsweetened coconut water, apple juice, or other fruit juices as the liquid in your baked goods to add a bit of sweetness—as well as moisture—to the final product. Applesauce, fruit purées, or vegan yogurt also work and greatly reduce the amount of sweetener needed. They also add moisture to your baked goods. Further, they can be used to replace all or part of the oil or nonhydrogenated margarine called for in a recipe.

Overall, gluten-free baked goods can dry out and get hard rather quickly, which is why the recipes in this chapter yield only small amounts, like 6 muffins, 8 biscuits, or 1 loaf. We recommend storing your baked goods in airtight containers or zipper-lock bags to keep them softer and fresher longer.

Beyond the logistics, let's talk about the exciting and unique recipes presented in this chapter. We start out with a savory muffin recipe, and then move on to the sweet stuff, like Yogurt and Berry Muffins, Banana-Date Bread, and—hold on to your hat—Chocolate, Chocolate Chip, and Raspberry Bread (which graces our cover). We share recipes for cornbread, biscuits, and a basic piecrust, too. Finally, we take the fear out of working with yeast by including several no-kneading-required recipes for hamburger buns, a multi-grain bread loaf, and pizza crust. Who says gluten free isn't heavenly?

Plant-Based Dietitian Recommends: As mentioned earlier, baking is a careful chemistry experiment—especially gluten-free vegan style. Thus, for the couple recipes in this chapter like the decadent Bettermilk Biscuits or Gluten-Free Piecrust where nonhydrogenated margarine is used, or for the others that include minimal oil, think of them as special treats to be used on occasion, since modifying them will drastically alter their integrity.

Soul Sisters Muffins

The Native American crop planting trio the "three sisters"—corn, beans, and squash—are regaled as the sustainers of life, and eating one of these lightly spiced, veggie-packed muffins gives you hours of sustainable energy.

Yield:	Prep time:	Cook time:	Serving size:
6 muffins	15 minutes	22 to 25 minutes	1 muffin

9 TB. medium-grind yellow cornmeal

6 TB. brown rice flour

4 TB. *chickpea/garbanzo bean flour*

1 TB. arrowroot

1 tsp. chili powder

1 tsp. aluminum-free baking powder

¾ tsp. baking soda

¼ tsp. sea salt

9 TB. canned butternut, pumpkin, or sweet potato purée

6 TB. plain or vanilla vegan yogurt

6 TB. soy milk or other nondairy milk

1 TB. maple syrup

3 TB. fresh or frozen cut corn kernels

3 TB. red bell pepper, diced

3 TB. zucchini, finely diced

3 TB. chopped fresh cilantro

2 TB. jalapeño pepper, ribs and seeds removed, and finely diced

1½ TB. raw pumpkin seeds

1. Preheat the oven to 400°F. Lightly oil 6 muffin cups, or line with paper liners, or use silicone muffin cups.

2. In a medium bowl, combine cornmeal, brown rice flour, chickpea/garbanzo bean flour, arrowroot, chili powder, baking powder, baking soda, and sea salt, and stir well.

3. In a small bowl, combine butternut purée, yogurt, soy milk, and maple syrup.

4. Pour wet ingredients into dry ingredients, and stir well to combine. Stir in corn, red bell pepper, zucchini, cilantro, and jalapeño pepper.

5. Fill the prepared muffin cups using a $\frac{1}{4}$ cup scoop or measuring cup. Sprinkle pumpkin seeds over top of each portioned muffin, and press them into batter gently with your fingers.

6. Bake for 22 to 25 minutes or until a toothpick inserted in the center comes out clean. Allow muffins to cool slightly in the pan and then transfer them to a rack to cool as desired.

7. Serve warm or at room temperature. Store extra muffins in an airtight plastic container or zipper-lock bag at room temperature.

Variation: For a sweeter version or **Golden Fruit and Nut Muffins,** replace the corn, red bell pepper, zucchini, and cilantro with $\frac{1}{3}$ cup raisins and $\frac{1}{3}$ cup dried cranberries, and also replace pumpkin seeds with 2 tablespoons finely chopped walnuts or pecans.

DEFINITION

Chickpea/garbanzo bean flour is made from dried chickpeas, which have been finely ground to a flourlike consistency. Due to its high protein content, this flour is great to substitute for wheat in gluten-free cooking and baking. Also referred to as besan or gram flour, it's often used in Middle Eastern, Indian, and African cuisines.

Yogurt and Berry Muffins

The combination of vegan yogurt and applesauce is used in these berry-dotted muffins to add moisture, some sweetness, and a bit of tanginess, as well as being a replacement for some of the oil typically called for in most muffin batters.

Yield:	Prep time:	Cook time:	Serving size:
6 muffins	5 to 7 minutes	18 to 22 minutes	1 muffin

1 cup plus 2 TB. Beverly's Baking Blend (recipe in Chapter 3) or Bob's Red Mill Gluten-Free All-Purpose Baking Flour

2 TB. turbinado sugar

1½ TB. arrowroot

2¼ tsp. aluminum-free baking powder

¼ tsp. plus ⅛ tsp. ground cinnamon

¼ tsp. plus ⅛ tsp. gluten-free xanthan gum

¼ tsp. sea salt

½ cup soy milk or other nondairy milk or apple juice

6 TB. plain or vanilla vegan yogurt

1½ TB. sunflower oil or other oil

1 tsp. alcohol-free vanilla extract

⅔ cup fresh or frozen blackberries, blueberries, raspberries, strawberries, or mixed berries of choice

1. Preheat the oven to 400°F. Lightly oil 6 muffin cups, or line with paper liners, or use silicone muffin cups.

2. In a medium bowl, combine Beverly's Baking Blend, turbinado sugar, arrowroot, baking powder, cinnamon, xanthan gum, and sea salt.

3. In a small bowl, whisk together soy milk, yogurt, sunflower oil, and vanilla extract.

4. Pour wet ingredients into dry ingredients, and whisk well to combine. Gently fold in berries.

5. Fill prepared muffin cups using a ¼ cup scoop or measuring cup.

6. Bake for 18 to 22 minutes or until a toothpick inserted in the center comes out clean. Allow muffins to cool slightly in the pan and then transfer to a rack to cool as desired.

7. Serve warm or at room temperature. Store extra muffins in an airtight plastic container or zipper-lock bag at room temperature.

Variation: You can easily change the flavor of your muffins by using other flavors of vegan yogurt, as well as by using different varieties of diced fruit, such as apples, cranberries, or peaches. For added crunch and protein, add a few tablespoons of chopped nuts to the batter, or sprinkle them over the top of the portioned muffins prior to baking.

CORNUCOPIA

Check the refrigerator case of your local grocery and natural foods stores to find several varieties of vegan yogurts, which are either soy-, rice-, or coconut-based. They come in a wide assortment of flavors such as plain, vanilla, or fruit-enhanced blends, such as mango, peach, raspberry, blueberry, lemon, lime, and orange, just to name a few. Vegan yogurts may be either unsweetened or sweetened with cane sugar, brown rice syrup, and fruit juices or purées.

Banana-Date Bread

Bananas and our Date Paste are great multitaskers as binding agents, oil replacements, and natural sweeteners in this lightly spiced, quick bread recipe.

Yield:	Prep time:	Cook time:	Serving size:
1 (8×4×2½-inch) loaf	8 to 10 minutes	35 to 40 minutes	1 slice

1⅓ cups brown rice flour

⅔ cup tapioca starch or arrowroot

½ cup chickpea/garbanzo bean flour

2 tsp. baking soda

2 tsp. ground cinnamon

1¼ tsp. ground ginger

1¼ tsp. gluten-free xanthan gum

½ tsp. sea salt

2 medium bananas, peeled and cut into 2-in. pieces

½ cup Date Paste (recipe in Chapter 8)

½ cup apple juice

¼ cup maple syrup

2 tsp. apple cider vinegar

2 tsp. alcohol-free vanilla extract

1. Preheat the oven to 375°F. Lightly oil a 8×4×2½-inch loaf pan, or use a silicone loaf pan.

2. In a medium bowl, combine brown rice flour, tapioca starch, chickpea/garbanzo bean flour, baking soda, cinnamon, ginger, xanthan gum, and sea salt, and whisk well.

3. In a blender or food processor fitted with an S blade, place bananas, Date Paste, apple juice, maple syrup, apple cider vinegar, and vanilla extract, and process for 1 minute. Scrape down the sides of the container with a spatula, and process for 1 or 2 more minutes or until smooth.

4. Pour wet ingredients into dry ingredients, and whisk well to combine.

5. Transfer batter into the prepared pan. Bake for 35 to 40 minutes or until a toothpick inserted in the center comes out clean. Allow loaf to cool slightly in the pan and then transfer to a rack to cool as desired.

6. Serve warm or at room temperature. Store loaf in an airtight plastic container or zipper-lock bag at room temperature.

Variation: Feel free to add ²⁄₃ cup fresh or frozen berries or vegan chocolate chips to the batter. You can also sprinkle ¼ cup finely chopped walnuts or other nuts or seeds over the top of the portioned batter prior to baking.

MEATLESS AND WHEATLESS

When using bananas in baked goods and desserts, it's best to use overly ripe bananas because they have a sweeter flavor. So when purchasing bananas for sweet treats, look for ones that feel soft when gently squeezed and have spotted or darkened peels, or allow unripe bananas to sit on your kitchen counter until they take on this appearance.

Chocolate, Chocolate Chip, and Raspberry Bread

Craving something ooey-gooey and chocolaty? Then bake up a loaf of this decadently rich, double-dosed chocolate quick bread, with melted bits of chocolate and tart and juicy red raspberries.

Yield:	Prep time:	Cook time:	Serving size:
1 (8×4×2½-inch) loaf	8 to 10 minutes	35 to 45 minutes	1 slice

¼ cup plus ⅔ cup water

2 TB. ground flaxseeds or flaxseed meal

⅔ cup brown rice flour

⅔ cup cocoa powder

½ cup arrowroot or tapioca starch

½ cup chickpea/garbanzo bean flour

2 tsp. aluminum-free baking powder

1 tsp. baking soda

1 tsp. gluten-free xanthan gum

½ tsp. sea salt

½ cup Prune Paste (variation in Chapter 8)

½ cup maple syrup

1½ tsp. alcohol-free vanilla extract

⅔ cup vegan gluten-free chocolate chips

⅔ cup fresh or frozen red raspberries

1. Preheat the oven to 375°F. Lightly oil a 8×4×2½-inch loaf pan, or use a silicone loaf pan.

2. In a medium bowl, combine ¼ cup water and ground flaxseeds, and let sit for 5 minutes.

3. In a large bowl, combine brown rice flour, cocoa powder, arrowroot, chickpea/garbanzo bean flour, baking powder, baking soda, xanthan gum, and sea salt, and whisk to combine.

4. Add Prune Paste, remaining ⅔ cup water, maple syrup, and vanilla extract to flaxseed mixture, and whisk well to combine.

5. Pour wet ingredients into dry ingredients, and whisk well to combine. Gently fold in chocolate chips and raspberries.

6. Transfer batter to the prepared pan. Bake for 35 to 45 minutes or until a tooth-pick inserted in the center comes out clean. Allow loaf to cool slightly in the pan, and transfer to a rack to cool as desired.

7. Serve warm or at room temperature, as a breakfast sweet treat or snack, or enjoy it later in the day as a dessert topped with your favorite nondairy ice cream or sorbet. Store loaf in an airtight plastic container or zipper-lock bag at room temperature.

Variation: If you have to avoid chocolate, replace the cocoa powder with carob powder, and the chocolate chips with carob chips. For **Black Forest Bread,** replace the raspberries with an equal amount of fresh or frozen cherries. For **Chocolate Walnut Brownie Bread,** omit the raspberries, increase the chocolate chips to 1 cup, and sprinkle ¼ cup finely chopped walnuts over the top of the portioned batter prior to baking.

> **CORNUCOPIA**
>
> You might be pleasantly surprised by how dried prunes and chocolate work together to boost the chocolaty flavor of this bread. For even more flavor, make your Prune Paste with coffee instead of water.

Country Cornbread

The addition of maple syrup helps enhance the natural sweetness of the cornmeal, and the nutritional yeast flakes play up its savory side in this comfort food classic.

Yield:	Prep time:	Cook time:	Serving size:
1 (9-inch) pan	5 minutes	22 to 25 minutes	1 piece

1¼ cups medium-grind yellow cornmeal

1 cup Beverly's Baking Blend (recipe in Chapter 3) or Bob's Red Mill Gluten-Free All-Purpose Baking Flour

1½ TB. aluminum-free baking powder

1 TB. nutritional yeast flakes

½ tsp. sea salt

1 cup soy milk or other nondairy milk

⅔ cup water

3 TB. sunflower or other oil

2 TB. maple syrup

1. Preheat the oven to 375°F. Lightly oil a 9-inch baking pan or use a silicone baking pan.

2. In a medium bowl, combine cornmeal, Beverly's Baking Blend, baking powder, nutritional yeast flakes, and sea salt.

3. In a small bowl, whisk together soy milk, water, sunflower oil, and maple syrup. Pour wet ingredients into dry ingredients, and stir well to combine.

4. Transfer batter to the prepared pan. Bake for 22 to 25 minutes or until a toothpick inserted in the center comes out clean. Allow to cool slightly, and cut into 8 or 9 pieces as desired. Serve warm or at room temperature.

Variation: Feel free to replace the yellow cornmeal with blue cornmeal.

MEATLESS AND WHEATLESS

When choosing cornmeal, opt for stone-ground cornmeal. This milling process retains more of the corn's beneficial hull and germ. Cornmeal is sold in various textural grinds. Use fine-grind as a replacement for all-purpose flour, and for breading or coating foods, choose medium-grind for the best-quality cornbread. Coarse-grind is commonly used for preparing polenta.

Bettermilk Biscuits

These biscuits are made with a *clabbered* soy milk mixture, which has a similar consistency to dairy-based buttermilk. Rather than use just margarine or oil, we've also added some vegan yogurt to help achieve the desired tenderness.

Yield:	Prep time:	Cook time:	Serving size:
8 (2-inch) biscuits	8 to 10 minutes	10 minutes	1 biscuit

6 TB. soy milk

1 TB. lemon juice

2 cups Bob's Red Mill Gluten-Free All-Purpose Baking Flour

1 TB. aluminum-free baking powder

½ tsp. gluten-free xanthan gum

½ tsp. sea salt

¼ cup nonhydrogenated margarine

¼ cup vegan yogurt

1. Preheat the oven to 400°F. Line a cookie sheet with parchment paper or a Silpat liner.

2. In a small bowl, combine soy milk and lemon juice. Set aside for 5 minutes to thicken.

3. In a medium bowl, combine Bob's Red Mill Gluten-Free All-Purpose Baking Flour, baking powder, xanthan gum, and sea salt.

4. Using a fork, work margarine into dry ingredients until mixture resembles coarse crumbs. Add soy milk mixture and yogurt, and stir just until combined. Using your hands, gather dough up into a ball in the bowl and knead dough lightly 5 times.

5. Transfer dough to the prepared cookie sheet. Using your hands, gently pat it out to 1-inch thickness. Cut dough with a 2-inch biscuit cutter or small glass, gathering up scraps and recutting them as necessary for a total of 8 biscuits. Space biscuits on the cookie sheet, either touching (for soft-sided biscuits) or 1 inch apart (for biscuits with lightly browned edges).

6. Bake for 10 to 12 minutes or until lightly browned on the bottom. Remove from the oven.

7. Serve hot, warm, or at room temperature as desired. Store biscuits in an airtight container at room temperature for up to 3 days.

Variation: For **Herbed Biscuits,** add 3 tablespoons chopped fresh herbs or 2 or 3 teaspoons dried herbs, such as basil, dill, or parsley to the dry ingredients. For **Cheesy Biscuits,** mix $1/3$ cup shredded Better Cheddar or Mellow Jack Cheese (recipes in Chapter 6) into the biscuit dough prior to shaping into a rectangle.

DEFINITION

Clabbering is done by combining soy milk (or other nondairy milk) with a little lemon juice or vinegar, which when left to sit for a few minutes, will curdle, causing the soy milk to sour and thicken slightly. Sometimes this mixture is affectionately referred to as soy buttermilk because it can be used as a measure-for-measure replacement for buttermilk in recipes.

Gluten-Free Hamburger Buns

These hamburger buns bake up light and soft, and we've even topped them with a few sesame seeds, just like their packaged, wheat-based counterparts.

Yield:	Prep time:	Cook time:	Serving size:
6 buns	10 minutes, plus 1 hour rise time	15 minutes	1 bun

$2\frac{1}{4}$ cups Bob's Red Mill Gluten-Free All-Purpose Baking Flour

$1\frac{1}{2}$ TB. nutritional yeast flakes

1 TB. gluten-free xanthan gum

1 tsp. agar powder

1 tsp. onion powder

1 tsp. sea salt

1 cup plus 2 TB. warm water (110°F to 115°F)

$1\frac{1}{2}$ tsp. unbleached cane sugar

1 (.25-oz.) pkg. or $2\frac{1}{4}$ tsp. rapid-rise active yeast

6 TB. cold water

3 TB. Ener-G Egg Replacer

3 TB. olive or other oil

$\frac{3}{4}$ tsp. apple cider vinegar

$1\frac{1}{2}$ tsp. raw sesame seeds

1. In a large bowl, combine Bob's Red Mill Gluten-Free All-Purpose Baking Flour, nutritional yeast flakes, xanthan gum, agar powder, onion powder, and sea salt, and set aside.

2. In a medium bowl, combine warm water, unbleached cane sugar, and yeast, and set aside for 5 to 7 minutes or until yeast is fully dissolved and mixture is very foamy.

3. In a small bowl, combine cold water and Ener-G Egg Replacer, and whisk vigorously for 1 minute or until very frothy (like beaten egg whites).

4. When yeast mixture is foamy, add egg replacer mixture, olive oil, and apple cider vinegar, and stir gently to combine. Add wet ingredients to dry ingredients, and stir well to combine (mixture will resemble a thick cake batter).

5. Line a large cookie sheet with parchment paper or a Silpat liner. Use a $\frac{1}{3}$ cup measuring cup to portion 6 hamburger buns onto the prepared cookie sheet, spacing them 3 inches apart. Dampen your hands with water, and press each portioned hamburger bun into a 4-inch-wide circle.

6. Sprinkle ¼ teaspoon sesame seeds over the top of each hamburger bun. Cover hamburger buns lightly with a clean towel (or plastic wrap), and let rise in a warm place for 1 hour.

7. Preheat the oven to 400°F.

8. After 1 hour, remove the towel (or plastic wrap) from hamburger buns. Bake for 15 minutes or until lightly browned on the bottom.

9. Split each hamburger bun in half and serve warm, at room temperature, or lightly toasted as desired. Store hamburger buns in an airtight container or zipper-lock bag at room temperature.

Variation: You can also top your hamburger buns with other seeds or use a mixture of seeds, such as black sesame seeds, hemp seeds, or poppy seeds. For a more golden-colored hamburger bun, replace ¼ cup Bob's Red Mill Gluten-Free All-Purpose Baking Flour with buckwheat flour. For **Gluten-Free Hot Dog Buns,** form each of the 6 portions into a 3×6-inch log instead and then cover, let rise, and bake in a similar manner.

MEATLESS AND WHEATLESS

One of the best places to let yeast-based baked goods rise is either on a sunny window sill or on a table or counter in direct sunlight.

Multi-Grain Sandwich Bread

This multipurpose loaf of bread, made with a combination of several gluten-free flours and starches, nutty flaxseeds, and some maple syrup for a bit of sweetness, has a nice, tender crumb inside and slightly chewy, golden brown crust.

Yield:	Prep time:	Cook time:	Serving size:
1 (9×5×2¾-inch) loaf	10 minutes, plus 1 hour rise time	40 to 45 minutes	1 slice

1 cup cornstarch

1 cup tapioca starch

⅔ cup chickpea/garbanzo bean flour

½ cup sorghum flour

¼ cup millet flour or quinoa flour

2 tsp. gluten-free xanthan gum

1½ tsp. agar powder

1 tsp. sea salt

¾ cup warm water (110°F to 115°F)

1½ TB. maple syrup

1 (.25-oz.) pkg. or 2¼ tsp. rapid-rise active yeast

9 TB. cold water

3 TB. ground flaxseeds or golden flaxseeds or flaxseed meal

¾ cup seltzer water

3 TB. olive or other oil

¾ tsp. apple cider vinegar

1. In a large bowl, combine cornstarch, tapioca starch, chickpea/garbanzo bean flour, sorghum flour, millet flour, xanthan gum, agar powder, and sea salt, and set aside.

2. In a medium bowl, combine warm water, maple syrup, and yeast, and set aside for 5 to 7 minutes or until yeast is fully dissolved and mixture is very foamy.

3. In a small bowl, combine cold water and flaxseeds, and let sit for 5 minutes.

4. When yeast mixture is foamy, add flaxseed mixture, seltzer water, olive oil, and apple cider vinegar, and stir gently to combine. Add wet ingredients to dry ingredients, and stir well to combine (mixture will be a very thick and soft bread dough).

5. Lightly oil a 9×5×2¾-inch loaf pan or use a silicone loaf pan. Spoon bread dough into the prepared loaf pan, and dampen your fingers with water and smooth the top. Cover bread dough lightly with a clean towel (or plastic wrap), and let rise in a warm place for 1 hour.

6. Preheat the oven to 400°F.

7. After 1 hour, remove the towel (or plastic wrap) from bread loaf. Bake for 40 to 45 minutes or until golden brown on top. Allow loaf to cool for 10 minutes in the pan and then loosen sides with a spatula, and transfer the loaf to a rack to cool completely.

8. Use a serrated bread knife to cut loaf into $\frac{1}{2}$-inch-thick slices as desired. Store loaf in an airtight container or zipper-lock bag at room temperature.

Variation: To further boost the nutrition level of this loaf, add 2 tablespoons nutritional yeast flakes to the dry ingredients. For added texture and flavor, once you've finished combining the wet and dry ingredients, mix in $\frac{1}{4}$ cup raw seeds or use a mixture of seeds, such as chia seeds, hemp seeds, pumpkin seeds, sunflower seeds, or sesame seeds.

> **AGAINST THE GRAIN**
>
> Flaxseeds have a high oil content and can become rancid rather quickly. For longer and safer storage, store your whole or freshly ground flaxseeds—as well as convenient packaged flaxseed meal—in airtight containers in your refrigerator or freezer.

Gluten-Free Piecrust

With a few gluten-free pantry staples, plus some margarine and a little cool water, you can quickly create your own gluten-free vegan piecrust suitable for both sweet and savory preparations.

Yield:	Prep time:
1 single (9-inch) piecrust	5 minutes, plus 30 minutes chill time

1½ cups Bob's Red Mill Gluten-Free All-Purpose Baking Flour	½ tsp. sea salt
½ tsp. aluminum-free baking powder	⅓ cup nonhydrogenated margarine
½ tsp. gluten-free xanthan gum	¼ cup cold water
	½ tsp. apple cider vinegar

1. In a medium bowl, combine Bob's Red Mill Gluten-Free All-Purpose Baking Flour, baking powder, xanthan gum, and sea salt.

2. Using a fork, work margarine into dry ingredients until it resembles coarse crumbs. Add cold water and apple cider vinegar, and stir until mixture just comes together to form a soft dough. Gather pastry dough into a ball, and flatten into a disc. Wrap disc in plastic wrap, and chill for 30 minutes or more.

3. For easier rolling, place chilled pastry dough disc between 2 (12×16-inch) pieces of parchment paper, and roll into a 12-inch circle for a 9-inch piecrust, or a 9- or 10-inch tart crust. Remove and discard top sheet of parchment paper.

4. Flip pastry dough into pie (or tart) pan, and remove and discard remaining parchment paper. Gently press pastry dough against the bottom and sides of pan. If using a pie pan, trim overhanging edge of pastry dough about 1 inch from the edge of the pie pan. Tuck excess pastry dough underneath, and flute edges as desired. Alternatively, if using a tart pan, after pressing pastry dough into the bottom and sides of the tart pan, simply trim and discard any overhanging edges.

5. Bake piecrust as per recipe instructions.

Variation: Feel free to roll the pastry dough into a 14-inch circle for use in making a free-form pie or galette. For a **Single Sweetened Gluten-Free Piecrust,** add either 2 tablespoons turbinado sugar to the dry ingredients, or replace 1 tablespoon cold water with an equal amount of maple syrup. For a **Double Gluten-Free Piecrust,** prepare your pastry dough using double the amounts of all the piecrust ingredients, divide it in half, wrap each half in plastic wrap, and chill for 30 minutes. After chilling, roll out each pastry dough half between sheets of parchment paper, and proceed as directed by the instructions for your particular recipe.

MEATLESS AND WHEATLESS

In this recipe, you'll notice that a little baking powder and apple cider vinegar is called for, which may seem strange at first glance. The baking powder gives the pastry dough some lift and makes it seem more tender. The vinegar also aids in the tenderness and flakiness, and helps the dough relax, making it easier to roll out, as well as shrink less during baking.

Pizza Crust

Our gluten-free pizza crust is made with a blend of brown rice, millet, and sorghum flours, potato and tapioca starch, and a bit of cornmeal.

Yield:	Prep time:	Cook time:
1 (12-inch) thick crust, 1 (14-inch) thin crust, or 1 (9×13-inch) rectangular crust	10 minutes, plus 1 hour rise time	15 to 20 minutes

1 cup warm water (110°F to 115°F)

1 TB. gluten-free brown rice syrup

1 (.25-oz.) pkg. or 2¼ tsp. rapid-rise active yeast

½ cup brown rice flour

½ cup millet flour

½ cup tapioca starch

⅓ cup potato starch

⅓ cup sorghum flour

2 TB. medium-grind yellow cornmeal, plus additional for dusting pan

1½ TB. nutritional yeast flakes

2 tsp. gluten-free xanthan gum

½ tsp. sea salt

1½ TB. olive oil

1. In a small bowl, combine warm water, brown rice syrup, and yeast, and set aside for 5 to 7 minutes or until yeast is fully dissolved and mixture is very foamy.

2. In a medium bowl, combine brown rice flour, millet flour, tapioca starch, potato starch, sorghum flour, cornmeal, nutritional yeast flakes, xanthan gum, and sea salt.

3. Lightly oil a large, round pizza pan or 9×13-inch baking pan. Evenly sprinkle a little cornmeal over the pan, and set aside.

4. Add yeast mixture and olive oil to dry ingredients, and stir well to combine.

5. Transfer pizza dough to the prepared pan. Using your hands, evenly spread out dough to the desired size and shape (either into a round 12-inch thick crust, a round 14-inch thin crust, or 9×13-inch rectangular crust). Cover crust lightly with a clean towel (or plastic wrap), and let rise in a warm place for 1 hour.

6. Preheat the oven to 450°F.

7. After 1 hour, remove the towel (or plastic wrap) from pizza crust. Top pizza crust with your choice of sauce and toppings. Bake for 15 to 20 minutes or until lightly browned on bottom and around edges.

Say "Cheese"!

In This Chapter

- Easy vegan Parmesan alternative
- Tofu-based ricotta
- Dairy-free cheese spreads, sauces, and blocks

One of the most commonly cited challenges to going full-fledged vegan is letting go of cheese. Americans have a love affair with cheese, and the thought of not having it in their daily diet is more than some people want to handle. Never fear, thanks to vegan cheeses!

We like to think of this chapter as our DIY Guide to Vegan Cheese Alternatives. In the following pages, we share ideas for making your own spicy herb–flavored, Parmesan-like sprinkles; tofu-based ricotta replacements; and cheesy-tasting sauces, spreads, and sliceable blocks. We've used wholesome ingredients in their preparation, like raw nuts, bell peppers, tofu, herbs and spices, and our secret vegan weapon for achieving a cheesy taste, the versatile nutritional yeast flakes.

You're bound to be especially impressed by the two block varieties of cheese in this chapter. Our Mellow Jack Cheese is a mild-flavored white variety, and the Better Cheddar has an orangey color reminiscent of the popular American and cheddar styles of cheese. These block styles are firm enough to be sliced or shredded and will even melt when heated, say, on a sandwich or pizza, or even on a batch of vegan nachos—yum!

Spicy Sprinkles

This vegan alternative to Parmesan cheese has a little kick to it, thanks to a generous combination of smoked paprika, cayenne, and chipotle chili powder.

Yield:	Prep time:	Serving size:
2 cups	2 or 3 minutes	1 tablespoon

½ cup raw walnuts

½ cup hemp seeds

1¼ cups *nutritional yeast flakes*

1 tsp. onion powder

1 tsp. smoked paprika or sweet paprika

½ tsp. cayenne

½ tsp. chipotle chili powder or chili powder

½ tsp. sea salt or Himalayan pink salt

1. In a food processor fitted with an S blade, combine walnuts and hemp seeds, and process for 1 or 2 minutes or until finely ground. Scrape down the sides of the container with a spatula.

2. Add nutritional yeast flakes, onion powder, smoked paprika, cayenne, chipotle chili powder, and sea salt, and process for 1 or 2 minutes or until well combined. Use as a condiment or to add flavor to sauces, salad dressings, gluten-free pasta, vegetables, and other dishes as desired. Store in an airtight container in the refrigerator for up to 2 months.

Variation: For a less spicy version, omit the cayenne, and use chili powder instead of chipotle chili powder. For **Italian Herb Sprinkles,** omit the smoked paprika, chipotle chili powder, and cayenne, and replace them with 1½ teaspoons dried basil, 1 teaspoon dried oregano, 1 teaspoon garlic powder or granules, and ½ teaspoon crushed red pepper flakes, or simply add 1 tablespoon Italian seasoning blend.

Tofu Ricotta

This tofu-based ricotta has a cheesy flavor thanks to a generous dose of nutritional yeast flakes, a bit of tanginess from lemon juice and miso, and a bit of savoriness from chopped fresh onion and garlic.

Yield:	Prep time:	Serving size:
2½ cups	3 to 5 minutes	¼ cup

1 lb. firm or extra-firm tofu

¼ cup nutritional yeast flakes

3 TB. lemon juice

2 TB. yellow onion or shallot, finely diced

2 TB. chopped fresh parsley

1½ TB. raw tahini

1½ TB. garlic, minced

2 tsp. mellow miso or other miso

1 tsp. onion powder

¼ tsp. freshly ground black pepper

Pinch freshly ground nutmeg

1. Using your fingers, crumble tofu into a medium bowl. Add nutritional yeast flakes, lemon juice, yellow onion, parsley, tahini, garlic, mellow miso, onion powder, pepper, and nutmeg, and mash with a fork until completely smooth. Alternatively, combine all ingredients in a food processor fitted with an S blade, and process for 1 or 2 minutes or until smooth.

2. Use tofu ricotta immediately or chill as desired. Use as a substitute for the traditional dairy-based version in lasagna, pizza, calzones, manicotti, stuffed shells, as well as your other favorite Italian dishes. Store in an airtight container in the refrigerator for up to 3 days.

Variation: For extra flavor, add 3 tablespoons chopped fresh basil, or 1 teaspoon each dried basil and oregano. To adapt this recipe to make **Cashew Ricotta,** soak ⅔ cup raw cashews in water for several hours or overnight, drain and rinse cashews, place

...rocessor, and process for 1 minute to finely grind. Add the remaining ...ients, but omit the chopped parsley, and process for an additional ...til completely smooth.

CORNUCOPIA

White, mellow, and chickpea miso have a light color and flavor, in comparison to red or hatcho miso, which have a reddish or dark brown color and a stronger, more robust flavor.

Raw Cashew Cheese Spread

Red bell pepper adds a bit of sweetness, in addition to aiding cayenne and smoked paprika with boosting the flavor and enhancing the color of this nut-based cheese spread.

Yield:	Prep time:	Serving size:
2 cups	5 minutes, plus 6 or more hours soak time	2 tablespoons

1 cup raw cashews

1 cup plus 2 TB. water

1 medium red bell pepper, ribs and seeds removed, and diced

3 large garlic cloves

Juice of 1 lemon

$\frac{1}{3}$ cup nutritional yeast flakes

$\frac{1}{2}$ tsp. *Himalayan pink salt* or sea salt

$\frac{1}{4}$ tsp. cayenne

$\frac{1}{4}$ tsp. smoked paprika or chili powder

1. In a small bowl, combine cashews and 1 cup water, and set aside to soak for 6 hours or overnight.

2. Drain off soaking water, rinse cashews, and drain again.

3. In a blender, place red bell pepper, garlic, and lemon juice, and process for 1 minute. Scrape down the sides of the container with a spatula, and process for 1 more minute or until smooth.

4. Add cashews, remaining 2 tablespoons water, nutritional yeast flakes, Himalayan pink salt, cayenne, and smoked paprika, and process for 1 minute. Scrape down the sides of the container with a spatula, and process for 1 more minute or until smooth.

5. Serve as a spread with raw veggies, fruit, gluten-free crackers or bread slices, or for wraps or sandwiches. Store cashew spread in an airtight container in the refrigerator for up to 1 week.

Variation: You can replace the cashews with macadamia nuts.

> **DEFINITION**
>
> **Himalayan pink salt** is a hand-mined salt derived from ancient sea salt deposits found in the Himalayan Mountains. Some consider it the purest variety of salt available. The salt crystals range in color from sheer white, to varying shades of pink, to deep red, due to its high mineral and iron content. Find it in grocery and natural foods stores, gourmet and specialty food shops, as well as online.

Cheesy Sauce

Vitamin B_{12}–rich nutritional yeast flakes impart a cheeselike flavor and combine nicely with orange bell pepper, chili powder, and smoked paprika to create the perfect orangey hue in this quick and easy sauce.

Yield:	Prep time:	Cook time:	Serving size:
$1\frac{1}{2}$ cups	3 to 5 minutes	3 to 5 minutes	$\frac{1}{4}$ cup

1 cup soy milk or other nondairy milk

$\frac{1}{2}$ cup orange bell pepper, diced

$\frac{1}{2}$ cup nutritional yeast flakes

2 TB. arrowroot

2 TB. raw tahini

2 tsp. Dijon mustard

$1\frac{1}{2}$ tsp. garlic powder

$\frac{3}{4}$ tsp. onion powder

$\frac{3}{4}$ tsp. sea salt

$\frac{3}{4}$ tsp. sweet paprika or smoked paprika

1. In a blender, place $\frac{2}{3}$ cup soy milk, orange bell pepper, nutritional yeast flakes, arrowroot, tahini, Dijon mustard, garlic powder, onion powder, sea salt, and sweet paprika, and blend for 1 or 2 minutes or until pieces of bell pepper are no longer visible. Scrape down the sides of the container with a spatula.

2. Add remaining $\frac{1}{3}$ cup soy milk, and blend for 15 more seconds.

3. Transfer mixture to a small saucepan, and cook over medium heat, whisking often, for 3 to 5 minutes or until thickened. Serve hot. Store leftovers in an airtight container in the refrigerator for up to 10 days.

Variation: For a more flavorful cheesy sauce, replace ½ cup soy milk with low-sodium vegetable broth. For a more yellow-colored cheese sauce, use yellow bell pepper instead of orange.

> **MEATLESS AND WHEATLESS**
>
> Transform this Cheesy Sauce into a pot of fondue by replacing the soy milk with a 12-ounce bottle of your favorite gluten-free beer, plus ¼ teaspoon chipotle chili powder to give it a little extra oomph! Serve with chunks of gluten-free breads, broccoli and cauliflower florets, and your other favorite dunking foods.

Better Cheddar

Orange bell peppers are used to flavor and tint this dairy-free cheese, but with the addition of *agar powder*, you're able to achieve a block of cheddarlike cheese you can slice or gently shred.

Yield:	Prep time:	Cook time:	Serving size:
1 (3-cup) block	5 minutes, plus 3 hours chill time	3 minutes	2 tablespoons shredded or 1 slice

1 medium orange bell pepper, ribs and seeds removed, and finely diced	1 tsp. garlic powder or garlic granules
⅔ cup raw cashews	1 tsp. onion powder
3 TB. nutritional yeast flakes	1 tsp. sweet paprika or smoked paprika
2 TB. raw tahini	1 tsp. sea salt
2 TB. lemon juice	1½ cups water
1 TB. Dijon mustard	2 TB. agar powder

1. In a food processor fitted with an S blade, combine orange bell pepper, cashews, nutritional yeast flakes, tahini, lemon juice, Dijon mustard, garlic powder, onion powder, sweet paprika, and sea salt, and process for 1 or 2 minutes or until pieces of bell pepper are no longer visible. Scrape down the sides of the container with a spatula.

2. In a small saucepan, combine water and agar powder, and cook over medium heat, stirring often, for 3 minutes or until it becomes a thickened, gel-like mixture. Remove from heat.

3. Add agar mixture to the food processor, and process for 1 minute. Scrape down the sides of the container with a spatula, and process for 30 more seconds.

4. Lightly oil a 3-cup plastic container. Pour mixture into container, cover, and chill for 3 hours or until firm.

5. Invert the container, and unmold cheese when ready to use. You can cut this cheese into slices for sandwiches, into cubes for eating as a snack, or gently shred it for use in recipes. Store cheese in its covered container in the refrigerator for up to 10 days.

Variation: For a smoky-flavored and slightly reddish-colored cheese, use a red bell pepper instead and also add ¹/₂ teaspoon chili powder or chipotle chili powder.

> **DEFINITION**
>
> **Agar powder** (a.k.a. agar-agar flakes) is odorless and tasteless and derived from a variety of seaweed. It can be used as a vegan replacement for gelatin (an animal-based by-product). You can find agar powder in natural foods stores and Asian specialty markets, and we recommend Telephone Brand.

Mellow Jack Cheese

Our version of Monterey Jack cheese is both sliceable and shredable, with a pale-yellow color and a mild nutty flavor, thanks to our Awesome Almond Milk.

Yield:	Prep time:	Cook time:	Serving size:
1 (3-cup) block	5 minutes, plus 3 hours chill time	3 minutes	2 tablespoons shredded or 1 slice

¹/₂ cup reserved almond pulp (from Awesome Almond Milk recipe in Chapter 4)

¹/₂ cup firm or extra-firm silken tofu

¹/₄ cup nutritional yeast flakes

¹/₄ cup lemon juice

2 TB. mellow miso

1 TB. Dijon mustard

1¹/₂ tsp. onion powder

1 tsp. garlic powder or garlic granules

1 tsp. sea salt

1¹/₂ cups Awesome Almond Milk (recipe in Chapter 4)

2 TB. agar powder

1. In a food processor fitted with an S blade, combine almond pulp, tofu, nutritional yeast flakes, lemon juice, mellow miso, Dijon mustard, onion powder,

garlic powder, and sea salt, and process for 1 or 2 minutes or until smooth. Scrape down the sides of the container with a spatula.

2. In a small saucepan, combine Awesome Almond Milk and agar powder, and cook over medium heat, stirring often, for 3 minutes or until mixture becomes extremely thick and saucelike. Remove from heat.

3. Add agar mixture to the food processor, and process for 1 minute. Scrape down the sides of the container with a spatula, and process for an additional 30 seconds.

4. Lightly oil a 3-cup plastic container. Pour mixture into the container, cover, and chill for 3 hours or until firm.

5. Invert the container, and unmold cheese for use. You can cut this cheese into slices for sandwiches, into cubes for eating as a snack, or gently shred it for use in recipes. Store cheese in its covered container in the refrigerator for up to 10 days.

Variation: To make a **Pepper Jack Cheese,** after blending in the agar mixture, stir in $\frac{1}{2}$ cup finely diced red bell pepper, 1 finely diced jalapeño pepper, $1\frac{1}{2}$ teaspoons Italian seasoning blend (or $\frac{1}{2}$ teaspoon each dried basil, oregano, and thyme), and $\frac{3}{4}$ teaspoon crushed red pepper flakes.

MEATLESS AND WHEATLESS

If you can't find agar powder, but you're able to track down agar-agar flakes, you can substitute them in these cheese recipes. However, you'll need to use a greater amount. To replace 1 teaspoon agar powder, use 2 tablespoons agar-agar flakes.

Snacks, Sauces, and Spreads

Now that you've learned a few basic staples for making your gluten-free vegan meals, you're ready to venture a little further with this new way of cooking and eating. In Part 3, we share recipes for tasty snacks, sauces, and spreads.

Snacking has become an integral part of our overly busy society. Actually, it's now commonly recommended that you eat several small meals and/or snacks throughout the day, rather than just three large ones. So we'll teach you how to make some quick, easy, and satisfying snacks for your everyday needs, as well as nutritious and delicious appetizers, protein-rich hummus and spreads, and tasty guacamole and salsas you can proudly serve at your next party or neighborhood potluck.

You'll also find a wide selection of sauces and accompaniments, both simple and complex, to add a bit of pizzazz to your daily meals!

Munchies and Taste-Bud Teasers

In This Chapter

- Nutritious things to nibble on
- Superspiced snacks
- Asian-inspired appetizers

Snacking can be good for you. Sometimes, hunger kicks in between meals and provides an opportunity to choose something light and nutritious. When it comes to snacking, you shouldn't just grab the first thing you get your hands on. Instead, when you find yourself with a case of the munchies, turn to one of the recipes in this chapter.

We may have cut the fat, but we didn't compromise in the flavor department—how does some Cajun seasoned popcorn or wasabi-coated chickpeas grab you? Throwing a party or going to a potluck? Impress your friends and family with some savory stuffed mushrooms, cheesy kale chips, and hand-rolled sushi or spring rolls.

You'll notice the use of Merlot in two recipes in this chapter. If you enjoy a good glass of wine or a hearty brew now and again, remember to look for a vegan selection. Animal products like fish swimbladders (called isinglass), egg albumin, and gelatin are commonly used to clarify wine and beer. Fortunately for us animal lovers, wine and beer can be made without these ingredients, and several companies do so. To identify which of the many products out there are refreshingly animal free, check out websites such as Barnivore (barnivore.com) and Vegans Are from Mars (vegans.frommars.org).

Raw Cauliflower "Shrimp" Cocktail

Pungent *prepared horseradish* is mixed with some ketchup, a little hot sauce, and black pepper to create a fiery cocktail sauce perfect for dipping.

Yield:	Prep time:	Serving size:
4 cups florets and ¾ cup cocktail sauce	5 minutes	1 cup florets and 3 tablespoons cocktail sauce

⅔ cup ketchup

2½ TB. prepared horseradish or 5 TB. fresh horseradish, finely grated

¼ tsp. hot pepper sauce

Pinch freshly ground black pepper or garlic pepper

1 large head cauliflower (approximately 4 cups), cut into florets

1. In a small bowl, combine ketchup, horseradish, hot pepper sauce, and pepper, and stir well.

2. Place bowl of cocktail sauce in the center of a large plate or platter. Place cauliflower florets around the bowl, and serve as either a snack or an appetizer.

Variation: If you like your cocktail sauce extra spicy, add an additional 1 or 2 tablespoons prepared horseradish as desired.

DEFINITION

Prepared horseradish is grated horseradish root that has been preserved in vinegar, or in the case of red horseradish, bottled with beet juice. It's usually sold in small glass jars or bottles in the refrigerated section of grocery and natural foods stores. However, be sure to check the ingredients label carefully to be sure it isn't actually horseradish sauce because that often contains eggs and/or dairy-based products.

Savory Kale Chips with Hemp and Flaxseeds

Once you taste these slightly salty and nutty-flavored crisp kale chips, you'll never look at a bunch of kale (as well as your favorite potato chips) the same way again!

Yield:	Prep time:	Cook time:	Serving size:
12 cups	20 to 25 minutes	4 to 6 hours if dehydrated or 25 to 30 minutes if baking	2 cups

2 large bunches green or purple kale (or a combination of both), stems removed

2 TB. wheat-free tamari or *Bragg Liquid Aminos*

2 TB. hemp oil or flax oil

2 TB. water

$\frac{1}{4}$ cup nutritional yeast flakes

2 tsp. garlic powder or garlic granules

$1\frac{1}{2}$ tsp. ground cumin

1 tsp. chili powder

$\frac{1}{2}$ tsp. cayenne or chipotle chili powder

$\frac{1}{2}$ tsp. Himalayan pink salt or sea salt

$\frac{1}{4}$ cup hemp seeds

$\frac{1}{4}$ cup finely ground flaxseeds or flaxseed meal

1. Evenly divide kale between 2 very large bowls. Over each bowlful of kale, drizzle 1 tablespoon tamari, 1 tablespoon hemp oil, and 1 tablespoon water. Using your hands, toss and gently massage kale leaves to evenly coat.

2. In a small bowl, combine nutritional yeast flakes, garlic powder, cumin, chili powder, cayenne, and Himalayan pink salt. Evenly divide between the 2 bowls, sprinkling mixture over kale. Using your hands, toss and gently massage kale leaves to evenly coat.

3. Over *each* bowlful of kale, sprinkle 2 tablespoons hemp seeds and 2 tablespoons flaxseeds, and again, toss and gently massage kale leaves to evenly coat.

4. To dehydrate, place kale leaves in a single layer on dehydrator racks (depending on the type of dehydrator you have, it will fill 4 or 5 racks). Dehydrate for 4 to 6 hours or until kale leaves are light and crispy. Alternatively, to bake, preheat the oven to 350°F. Line 2 cookie sheets with parchment paper or Silpat liners. Working in batches, place kale leaves in a single layer on the prepared cookie

sheets, and bake for 15 minutes. Remove from the oven, flip over kale leaves, and bake for 10 to 15 more minutes or until kale leaves are light and crispy. Repeat procedure with remaining kale leaves as needed.

5. Enjoy kale chips as a snack, or lightly crush them up over popcorn, gluten-free pasta, or salads as desired. Store kale chips in an airtight container at room temperature for up to 5 days.

Variation: For **Cheesy Kale Chips,** in a medium bowl, whisk together $1\frac{1}{2}$ cups Raw Cashew Cheese Spread (recipe in Chapter 6) and $\frac{1}{3}$ cup water. Evenly divide cheese spread mixture between the 2 bowls of kale. Using your hands, toss and gently massage kale leaves to evenly coat. Dehydrate or bake kale leaves as described.

Plant-Based Dietitian Recommends: Substitute 2 tablespoons vegetable broth or water for the hemp or flax oil. If baking (instead of dehydrating), bake for 15 minutes. Remove from the oven, flip over kale leaves, and bake for 5 to 10 more minutes or until kale leaves are light and crispy.

DEFINITION

Bragg Liquid Aminos is made from soybeans and water and has a salty, rich flavor similar to tamari or soy sauce. It's commonly used as a condiment and flavor enhancer by raw foodists because it contains large amounts of dietary essential and nonessential amino acids. Bragg Liquid Aminos is gluten free, and you can find it alongside tamari in most grocery and natural foods stores.

Cajun Popcorn

This popcorn is spiced up with a homemade Cajun seasoning blend of fragrant oregano and thyme combined with chili and garlic powders.

Yield:	Prep time:	Cook time:	Serving size:
8 cups	1 to 2 minutes	5 minutes	2 cups

2½ tsp. low-sodium vegetable broth or water

1½ tsp. olive oil

1½ TB. nutritional yeast flakes

1 tsp. chili powder

¾ tsp. garlic powder or garlic granules

¾ tsp. dried oregano

¾ tsp. dried thyme

½ tsp. sea salt

8 cups plain popped popcorn

1. Place a small saucepan over medium heat. Add vegetable broth, olive oil, nutritional yeast flakes, chili powder, garlic powder, oregano, thyme, and sea salt, and cook, stirring often, for 1 or 2 minutes or until mixture is fragrant and warm through. Remove from heat.

2. In a large bowl, place popcorn. Drizzle warm, seasoned vegetable broth mixture over popcorn, and toss gently to evenly coat popcorn. Serve immediately.

Variation: For extra-spicy popcorn, add ¼ teaspoon cayenne or chipotle chili powder to the Cajun seasoning blend. You can vary the flavor of your popcorn by using other seasonings, such as curry powder, Italian seasoning blend, or just use garlic powder alone.

Plant-Based Dietitian Recommends: Substitute ½ cup vegetable broth or water for the oil.

CORNUCOPIA

Popcorn was first cultivated and consumed by Native Americans, and most of the popcorn sold worldwide is still grown in the United States. In fact, five Midwestern cities claim to be the "Popcorn Capital of the World": Ridgway, Illinois; Valparaiso, Indiana; Van Buren, Indiana; Schaller, Iowa; Marion, Ohio; and North Loup, Nebraska.

Ginger-Wasabi Roasted Chickpeas

The slightly sweet, salty, and exotic flavor combination of this tasty snack was inspired by crunchy wasabi-coated peas, which are sold in packages by themselves or as part of an Asian-style snack mix.

Yield:	Prep time:	Cook time:	Serving size:
2 to 2½ cups	18 to 20 minutes	35 to 40 minutes	¼ cup

2 (15-oz.) cans chickpeas, drained and rinsed

2 TB. wheat-free tamari

2 TB. gluten-free brown rice syrup

4 tsp. toasted sesame oil

2 TB. *wasabi powder*

2 tsp. ground ginger

1½ tsp. garlic powder or garlic granules

½ tsp. dry mustard

1. Place chickpeas in an even layer on a clean kitchen towel or paper towel, and allow to air dry for 15 minutes.

2. Preheat the oven to 425°F. Line a large cookie sheet with parchment paper or a Silpat liner.

3. Transfer chickpeas to a medium bowl. Add tamari, brown rice syrup, toasted sesame oil, wasabi powder, ginger, garlic powder, and dry mustard, and stir well to evenly coat chickpeas.

4. Transfer chickpea mixture to the prepared cookie sheet, and spread them into a single layer. Bake for 35 to 40 minutes, shaking the cookie sheet every 10 minutes to ensure even baking, or until chickpeas are dry and slightly crunchy. Remove from the oven.

5. Serve at room temperature. Store chickpeas in an airtight container at room temperature for up to 5 days.

Variation: For **Mediterranean Lemon-Herb Chickpeas,** replace the wasabi-tamari mixture with 2 tablespoons maple syrup, 4 teaspoons olive oil, 1 tablespoon lemon juice, 2 teaspoons tamari, 1 tablespoon herbes de Provence or dried rosemary, 1 tablespoon garlic powder or garlic granules, and 1½ teaspoons smoked paprika or sweet paprika, and bake chickpeas as described.

Plant-Based Dietitian Recommends: Omit the oil. Use 2 teaspoons sesame seeds, if desired, for flavoring.

> **DEFINITION**
>
> **Wasabi powder** is made from a variety of green horseradish grown only in Japan and is highly valued for its fiery flavor. Equal parts of wasabi powder are combined with warm water to make wasabi paste, a condiment often used in Asian cuisine, especially sushi. It can also be used to flavor sauces, salad dressings, mayonnaise, gluten-free pasta, mashed potatoes, and other vegetable dishes.

Stuffed Merlot Mushrooms

These savory stuffed morsels are filled with a mixture of freshly made breadcrumbs, aromatic vegetables, and lacinato kale, which we've infused with some herbs, vegetable broth, and marvelous Merlot wine.

Yield:	Prep time:	Cook time:	Serving size:
16 mushrooms	15 to 20 minutes	20 to 25 minutes	2 mushrooms

2 slices Multi-Grain Sandwich Bread (recipe in Chapter 5)

16 large crimini mushrooms

$\frac{1}{2}$ cup red onion, finely diced

$\frac{1}{2}$ cup celery, finely diced

$\frac{1}{3}$ cup green onion, thinly sliced

$\frac{1}{4}$ cup low-sodium vegetable broth

$1\frac{1}{4}$ cups lacinato (Italian) kale, washed well, stems removed, and finely chopped

$1\frac{1}{2}$ TB. garlic, minced

$1\frac{1}{4}$ tsp. dried basil

$1\frac{1}{4}$ tsp. dried thyme

$\frac{1}{2}$ tsp. freshly ground black pepper or garlic pepper

3 TB. Merlot or other red wine

3 TB. nutritional yeast flakes

1 TB. wheat-free tamari

3 TB. chopped fresh parsley (preferably Italian flat-leaf parsley)

1. In a food processor fitted with an S blade, place Multi-Grain Sandwich Bread slices, and process for 1 minute or until you get fine crumbs. Transfer breadcrumbs to a large plate, and set aside to dry out while preparing remaining filling ingredients.

2. Remove stems from crimini mushrooms, set caps aside, and finely chop stems.

3. Place a large, nonstick skillet over medium heat. Add mushroom stems, red onion, celery, green onion, and vegetable broth, and cook, stirring often, for 5 minutes. Add kale, garlic, basil, thyme, and pepper, and cook, stirring often, for 1 more minute.

4. Add Merlot and cook, stirring often, for 3 to 5 more minutes or until liquid is all absorbed. Remove from heat.

5. Preheat the oven to 375°F. Lightly oil a 9×13-inch baking pan.

6. Measure out ¾ cup breadcrumbs (save any extra for use in another recipe). Add them to vegetable mixture, along with nutritional yeast flakes, tamari, and parsley, and stir well to combine. Fill each crimini mushroom cap with a heaping 1 tablespoonful filling mixture, and place into the prepared pan.

7. Bake for 22 to 25 minutes or until crimini mushrooms are tender. Remove from the oven, and serve hot.

Variation: For a breadcrumb-free version, replace the breadcrumbs with ¾ cup cooked quinoa. For an alcohol-free version, replace the Merlot with additional vegetable broth.

MEATLESS AND WHEATLESS

Unless you're using dried mushrooms, you don't want to soak mushrooms to clean them. Much like a sponge, they'll soak up a lot of water, which will give them a mushy texture. Some chefs prefer to simply wipe off mushrooms with a damp towel to remove any debris or dirt. Others favor the combination technique of quickly cleaning them under running cold water, while gently rubbing the caps and stems with their fingers to remove any clinging dirt.

Tasty Thai Spring Rolls

Crunchy fresh veggies and lightly seasoned thin rice noodles are rolled in rice papers to create these fantastic rolls, perfect served with Miso-Peanut Sauce for a truly Thai experience.

Yield:	Prep time:	Cook time:	Serving size:
6 spring rolls	20 to 25 minutes	2 or 3 minutes	1 spring roll

1 oz. rice vermicelli noodles (about $\frac{1}{2}$ to $\frac{2}{3}$ cup cooked noodles)

1 tsp. wheat-free tamari

1 tsp. toasted sesame oil

1 tsp. sesame seeds, black sesame seeds, or hemp seeds

$\frac{1}{4}$ tsp. crushed red pepper flakes

3 large leaves red-tipped loose-leaf lettuce, washed well, patted dry, and cut in $\frac{1}{2}$

$\frac{1}{2}$ cup carrots, cut into matchsticks

$\frac{1}{2}$ cup cucumber, cut into matchsticks

$\frac{1}{2}$ cup red bell pepper, cut into matchsticks

1 cup Fresh and Flavorful Sprouts using mung beans (recipe in Chapter 10)

$\frac{1}{2}$ cup fresh cilantro leaves

6 (8- or 9-in.) round rice papers

1 batch Miso-Peanut Sauce (recipe in Chapter 9)

1. Submerge rice noodles in a bowlful of warm water for 8 to 10 minutes or until soft and clear. Drain noodles, cut into 2-inch pieces, and place in a medium bowl. Add tamari, toasted sesame oil, sesame seeds, and crushed red pepper flakes, and toss well to evenly coat noodles.

2. On a large platter or cookie sheet, in separate sections, place lettuce leaves, carrots, cucumber, red bell pepper, Fresh and Flavorful Sprouts using mung beans, and cilantro leaves.

3. Fill a 9-inch round pie pan with warm water. Working with 1 rice paper at a time, submerge it in water, and leave for 10 to 20 seconds or until soft and pliable. Remove rice paper from water, and place on a large plate or work surface.

4. To assemble each spring roll, place 1 lettuce leaf horizontally in center of rice paper. Top with $\frac{1}{6}$ of rice noodles. Then, horizontally in rows, place $\frac{1}{6}$ of each: carrots, cucumber, red bell pepper, and Fresh and Flavorful Sprouts using mung beans. Top with a few cilantro leaves.

5. Fold bottom edge of rice paper up over filling, fold side edges of rice paper toward center, and roll up from the bottom edge, as tightly as possible to enclose filling.

6. Place spring roll, seam side down, on a large plate. Assemble remaining rice papers in a similar manner. For faster assembly, soak 1 rice paper while you fill and roll another.

7. Cut each spring roll diagonally in half lengthwise and serve with Miso-Peanut Sauce. Store spring rolls in an airtight container or individually wrapped in plastic wrap in the refrigerator for up to 3 days.

Variation: You can replace the cucumber with thin slices of Hass avocado.

Plant-Based Dietitian Recommends: Omit the oil.

CORNUCOPIA

You can find rice papers in Asian markets, as well as the Asian foods aisle of most grocery and natural foods stores. If you can't track them down, use gluten-free tortillas, such as brown rice or hemp, instead.

Smoky Tempeh Sushi Rolls

This sassy vegan sushi combines warm, smoked flavors with crisp and refreshing sweet bell peppers and carrots for a tasty twist on standard veggie sushi rolls.

Yield:	Prep time:	Serving size:
4 rolls	10 minutes	1 roll

4 sheets nori

$\frac{1}{2}$ cup cooked brown rice

8 slices Smoky Tempeh Un-Bacon (recipe in Chapter 12), each slice cut in $\frac{1}{2}$ lengthwise (16 thin slices)

$\frac{1}{4}$ cup Hass avocado, peeled, pitted, and thinly sliced

$\frac{1}{2}$ cup red bell pepper, *julienned*

$\frac{1}{2}$ cup carrots, julienned

$\frac{1}{4}$ cup Fresh and Flavorful Sprouts using fenugreek (recipe in Chapter 10)

1 TB. sesame seeds or gomasio

$\frac{1}{2}$ TB. pickled ginger (optional)

1 tsp. wheat-free tamari (optional)

$\frac{1}{2}$ tsp. wasabi paste (optional)

1. In an assembly line fashion, on a large, dry work surface, align 4 nori sheets. Gently spoon 2 tablespoons brown rice onto $\frac{1}{2}$ of each nori sheet, patting down for even placement from top to bottom.

2. To fill each nori sheet, add, in this order, 2 slices Smoky Tempeh Un-Bacon, 1 tablespoon Hass avocado, 2 tablespoons each red bell pepper and carrots, and 1 tablespoon Fresh and Flavorful Sprouts using fenugreek. Sprinkle $\frac{1}{4}$ teaspoon sesame seeds over the top.

3. With each nori sheet, turn nori so ingredient side is facing you and empty nori is facing away from you. Fold bottom edge of nori roll up over filling, and roll up from the bottom edge as tightly as possible to enclose filling. Repeat procedure for remaining nori sheets.

4. With a sharp knife, slice each nori roll horizontally into 6 even pieces. Serve immediately with pickled ginger, tamari, and wasabi paste.

Variation: Try shredded cabbage and thinly sliced tomatoes in place of the red bell pepper, carrots, and Fresh and Flavorful Sprouts using fenugreek for a nori-style avocado BLT.

DEFINITION

Julienne is a French word meaning "to slice into very thin pieces." Here's how: after washing and peeling your vegetable, cut a flat surface on each of the vegetable's 4 sides, making a rectangle shape. Next, cut ⅛-inch slices through the vegetable. Finally, stack the rectangles flat on top of one another and repeat the ⅛-inch slices again, until you have thin, matchsticklike strips.

Olé Noritos

These noritos are creamy and crispy, cool and spicy all at the same time—a fiesta all wrapped up in a nori sheet!

Yield:	Prep time:	Serving size:
4 rolls	5 minutes	1 roll

4 sheets nori

4 TB. Spicy Cilantro-Lime Black Bean Spread (recipe in Chapter 8)

4 TB. Whoo-Pea Guacamole (recipe in Chapter 8)

¼ cup cucumber, julienned

¼ cup jicama, julienned

½ TB. chopped fresh cilantro

2 TB. store-bought salsa or Sausalito Salsa (recipe in Chapter 8)

1. In an assembly line fashion, on a large, dry work surface, align 4 nori sheets. Gently and evenly spread 1 tablespoon Spicy Cilantro-Lime Black Bean Spread on ½ of each nori sheet. Spoon 1 tablespoon Whoo-Pea Guacamole on top of bean spread.

2. To fill each nori sheet, add, in this order, ¼ each of julienned cucumber, jicama, and cilantro, followed by ½ tablespoon salsa.

3. Tightly roll each nori sheet from bottom to top to enclose filling ingredients. Serve immediately.

CORNUCOPIA

Nori sheets provide a flavorful, nutrient-rich kick. You can find them in most grocery stores, natural foods stores, or Asian specialty markets.

Delectable Dips and Spreads

In This Chapter

- Tasty vegan pâtés
- Out-of-the-ordinary bean-based dips and spreads
- So-good salsas

Dips, spreads, and salsas have a lot to offer. Consider the recipes in this chapter for not only toppings and teasers, but as inspiration for entire meals. Instead of using the typical bland, high-fat, low-nutrient varieties (think ketchup, mayo, and sour cream), tempt your taste buds with spice, flare, and flavor. It's a win-win situation when you mix flavor with quality nutrition.

Dried dates and other fruits can serve as sweeteners and even replace oil in baked goods. In the following recipes, we show you how decadent and moist puréed dried fruit can make a finished product. Wait until you sample Banana-Date Bread made with Date Paste and Chocolate, Chocolate Chip, and Raspberry Bread baked with Prune Paste (recipes in Chapter 5).

If you previously enjoyed eating pâté, you're in luck. We've come up with two vegan pâtés. One is made with nuts and other all-raw ingredients, and the other showcases the complex flavors of tempeh and crimini mushrooms.

Put on some lively Latino music, head to the kitchen, and start chopping. In no time, you'll have your own freshly made salsa. Olé!

Date Paste

Melt-in-your-mouth date paste can sweeten beverages, sauces, salad dressings, raw food dishes, desserts, and baked goods. You can also use it as a jamlike spread on gluten-free bread or crackers.

Yield:	Prep time:	Serving size:
½ cup	2 or 3 minutes, plus 30 minutes or more soak time	1 tablespoon

½ cup dried dates (about 6 to 8), pitted	5 TB. water

1. In a small bowl, combine dates and water, and set aside to soak for 30 minutes or until dates are very soft.

2. Transfer dates and water to a food processor fitted with an S blade, and process for 1 minute. Scrape down the sides of the container with a spatula, and process for 1 more minute or until a smooth purée. Store date paste in an airtight container in the refrigerator for up to 1 week.

Variation: For a sweeter date paste, replace the water with apple or orange juice. You can use this same procedure to make other dried fruit-based pastes. For **Apricot Paste,** use ½ cup dried apricots (about 8) and 5 tablespoons water or orange juice. For **Prune Paste,** use ½ cup dried pitted prunes (about 8) and 5 tablespoons water or coffee. For **Raisin Paste,** use ⅔ cup raisins and 5 tablespoons water or orange juice.

MEATLESS AND WHEATLESS

Our favorite dried dates to use in recipes are medjool dates, which are often referred to as "the king of dates" due to their rather large, plump size. But medjools can be quite expensive, so we also recommend using deglet noor or honey dates.

Veggie and Nut Pâté

This mock salmon pâté blends pistachios, sunflower seeds, carrots, and other fresh veggies with fragrant and warming spices like curry powder, cumin, and cayenne, and a bit of *powdered kelp* for a taste of the sea.

Yield:	Prep time:	Serving size:
1¼ to 1½ cups	10 minutes, plus 6 or more hours soak time	2 tablespoons

½ cup water

¼ cup raw pistachios

¼ cup raw sunflower seeds

1 large carrot, diced (about ¾ cup)

3 TB. celery, diced

3 TB. red onion, diced

2 TB. chopped fresh parsley

1 large garlic clove

¼ cup orange juice

1 TB. raw tahini

½ tsp. powdered kelp

½ tsp. ground coriander

½ tsp. ground cumin

½ tsp. curry powder

¼ tsp. Himalayan pink salt or sea salt

¹⁄₁₆ tsp. cayenne

1 tsp. hemp seeds or gomasio (optional)

1. In a small bowl, combine water, pistachios, and sunflower seeds, and set aside to soak for 6 hours or overnight.

2. Drain off soaking water, rinse pistachios and sunflower seeds, and drain again.

3. Transfer pistachios and sunflower seeds to a food processor fitted with an S blade, and process for 1 minute or until finely ground. Add carrot, celery, red onion, parsley, and garlic, and process for 1 or 2 minutes or until finely ground. Scrape down the sides of the container.

4. Add orange juice, tahini, powdered kelp, coriander, cumin, curry powder, Himalayan pink salt, and cayenne, and process for 1 or 2 minutes or until smooth. Scrape down the sides of the container, and process for 30 more seconds.

5. Transfer to a small bowl, and sprinkle hemp seeds (if using) over the top for garnish. Serve with celery sticks, slices of zucchini or yellow summer squash, or thin slices of gluten-free bread or crackers. Store pâté in an airtight container in the refrigerator for up to 5 days.

Variation: For a more fishy flavor, replace the powdered kelp with $^1/_2$ teaspoon dulse flakes. For an even more exotic-flavored pâté, replace the ground coriander with garam masala.

> **DEFINITION**
>
> **Powdered kelp** is made from cleaned and sun-dried kelp, a type of seaweed (or sea vegetable) that provides your body with sources of vitamin K, folate, magnesium, and calcium, as well as iodine, which aids in healthy thyroid function. A little powdered kelp or other sea vegetables added to your dishes imparts a slightly fishy flavor, which is why they're commonly added to mock fish dishes.

Tempeh and Mushroom Pâté

The savory flavor of this meat-free pâté is achieved by blending a mixture of cooked tempeh, crimini mushrooms, and shallots, which have been enhanced with a little red wine, fragrant *herbes de Provence*, and miso.

Yield:	Prep time:	Cook time:	Serving size:
2 cups	10 minutes	10 minutes	2 tablespoons

1 (8-oz.) pkg. tempeh

6 oz. crimini mushrooms or white button mushrooms, roughly chopped (about $1^1/_2$ cups)

1 cup red onion or shallots, diced

6 TB. low-sodium vegetable broth

1 TB. garlic, minced

$1^1/_2$ tsp. herbes de Provence

$^1/_4$ cup Merlot or other red wine

$1^1/_2$ TB. wheat-free tamari

$^1/_4$ tsp. freshly ground black pepper or garlic pepper

1 tsp. mellow miso or other miso

1. Place a large, nonstick skillet over medium heat. Using your fingers, crumble tempeh into the skillet. Add crimini mushrooms, red onion, and 4 tablespoons vegetable broth, and cook, stirring often, for 5 minutes.

2. Add garlic, herbes de Provence, and remaining 2 tablespoons vegetable broth, and cook, stirring often, for 2 more minutes.

3. Stir in Merlot, tamari, and pepper. Reduce heat to low, and cook, stirring often, for 2 more minutes or until all liquid is absorbed. Remove from heat and set aside to cool for 10 minutes.

4. Transfer tempeh mixture to a food processor fitted with an S blade. Add mellow miso, and process for 1 or 2 minutes or until smooth. Transfer pâté to a small bowl or dish, cover, and chill for 1 hour or more to allow flavors to blend.

5. Serve pâté with thin slices of gluten-free bread or crackers. Store pâté in an airtight container in the refrigerator for up to 1 week.

Variation: For added flavor, replace 1 tablespoon Merlot with an equal amount of balsamic vinegar. If you can't find herbes de Provence, you can replace it with $\frac{1}{2}$ teaspoon dried basil, $\frac{1}{2}$ teaspoon dried oregano, and $\frac{1}{2}$ teaspoon dried rosemary, which has been crushed a bit with your fingers.

DEFINITION

Herbes de Provence, or Provençal herbs, is a mixture of dried herbs commonly found growing in the Provence region of southeastern France and, therefore, used in the cuisine of that area. This aromatic blend of herbs typically consists of bay leaves, basil, chervil, fennel, marjoram, oregano, tarragon, thyme, summer savory, and rosemary. American mixes also often include lavender.

Garnet Yam Hummus

This vivid and elegant twist on hummus will tantalize your taste buds with its delicately warm, robust flavors. Serve it as a dip with raw veggies, rice cakes, or corn thins, or as a spread on gluten-free tortillas, nori wraps, or Multi-Grain Sandwich Bread.

Yield:	Prep time:	Serving size:
2½ cups	10 minutes	¼ cup

1 (15-oz.) can chickpeas, drained and rinsed

1 cup baked garnet yam or other yam or sweet potato

½ cup lemon juice

2 TB. nutritional yeast flakes

2 large garlic cloves

2 tsp. sweet paprika or smoked paprika

½ tsp. cayenne

½ tsp. chipotle chili powder

¼ tsp. ground cumin

Pinch sea salt

1. In a food processor fitted with an S blade, combine chickpeas, garnet yam, lemon juice, nutritional yeast flakes, garlic, sweet paprika, cayenne, chipotle chili powder, cumin, and sea salt, and process for 1 or 2 minutes or until smooth. Scrape down the sides of the container with a spatula, and process for 30 more seconds.

2. Transfer mixture to an airtight container. Serve immediately with raw veggies, rice cakes, or other options as desired. Store hummus in an airtight container in the refrigerator for up to 3 or 4 days.

Variation: You can replace the baked yam with 1 cup canned sweet potato or butternut squash purée. If you prefer a less smoky flavor, omit the chipotle chili powder.

CORNUCOPIA

Much controversy surrounds the identity of the yam versus the sweet potato. In the United States, yams are most likely sweet potatoes and have a moist, orange flesh. There are botanical and nutritional distinctions between the two, and it's difficult to find a real yam outside South America, Africa, or the Caribbean. Both of these tubers are nutrient dense with a slightly sweet flavor, so freely enjoy them regardless of their title.

Spicy Cilantro-Lime Black Bean Spread

Savor this flavor explosion where tangy meets hot and earthy meets zesty. Sun-dried tomato adds saltiness to the fresh cilantro and sour lime.

Yield:	Prep time:	Serving size:
1 ½ cups	10 minutes	¼ cup

½ cup whole sun-dried tomatoes

1 (15-oz.) can black beans, drained and rinsed

½ cup water

½ cup fresh cilantro leaves, tightly packed

¼ cup lime juice

2 TB. nutritional yeast flakes

1 tsp. lime zest

1 tsp. chili powder

½ tsp. ground cumin

¼ tsp. cayenne

1. In a food processor fitted with an S blade, place sun-dried tomatoes, and process for 2 minutes or until finely minced.

2. Add black beans, water, cilantro, lime juice, nutritional yeast flakes, lime zest, chili powder, cumin, and cayenne, and process for 1 or 2 minutes or until smooth. Scrape down the sides of the container with a spatula, and process for 30 to 60 more seconds.

3. Transfer mixture to an airtight container. Serve on corn tortillas with fresh romaine lettuce and tomatoes or as a spread for Olé Noritos (recipe in Chapter 7). Store bean spread in an airtight container in refrigerator for up to 3 or 4 days.

Variation: You can replace the black beans with an equal amount of pinto beans. Also, feel free to replace lime juice and zest with lemon juice and zest.

MEATLESS AND WHEATLESS

Sun-dried tomatoes can provide a pungent, slightly salty flavor to your dishes. You can grind them up in a food processor and use as a salt replacement for soups, spreads, salad dressings, and casseroles.

Whoo-Pea Guacamole

Adding sweet green peas (or other green-colored legumes or vegetables) boosts the nutritional value and vibrant color, as well as greatly reduces the fat content of this tortilla chip sidekick.

Yield:	Prep time:	Serving size:
2½ cups	8 to 10 minutes	¼ cup

1 (10-oz.) pkg. frozen peas, slightly thawed

1 medium Hass avocado, peeled, pitted, and diced

Juice of 1 lime

1 TB. garlic, minced

1 large Roma tomato, seeds removed and diced

⅓ cup red onion, finely diced

1 jalapeño pepper or serrano chile pepper, ribs and seeds removed, and finely diced

¼ cup chopped fresh cilantro

½ tsp. sea salt

¼ tsp. chipotle chili powder or chili powder

¼ tsp. fresh ground black pepper

1. In a food processor fitted with an S blade, place thawed peas, and process for 1 minute. Scrape down the sides of the container with a spatula, and process for 1 or 2 more minutes or until smooth.

2. In a medium bowl, combine Hass avocado, lime juice, and garlic. Using a potato masher or a fork, mash mixture as smooth or chunky as desired.

3. Stir in peas. Add Roma tomato, red onion, jalapeño pepper, cilantro, sea salt, chipotle chili powder, and pepper, and stir well to combine.

4. Serve as a snack or appetizer with raw veggies or tortilla chips; use as spread for nori rolls, wraps, or sandwiches; or use as a topping for tacos, burritos, or other Mexican dishes. Store covered with plastic wrap in an airtight container in the refrigerator for up to 3 days.

Variation: You can replace the peas with an equal amount of thawed shelled edamame or broccoli florets or 1 (15-ounce) can cannellini or navy beans. For extra flavor, add 1 tablespoon nutritional yeast flakes.

MEATLESS AND WHEATLESS

If you aren't serving this guacamole immediately, place a piece of plastic wrap directly on the surface of the guacamole and press it down gently to remove any excess air. This helps prevent browning.

Sausalito Salsa

Made with all fresh ingredients, this salsa is literally bursting at the seams with vibrant color and fresh, earthy flavors. It's a great way to showcase all the great summer vegetables available at your local farmers' market.

Yield:	Prep time:	Serving size:
4 cups	10 to 15 minutes	¼ cup

1½ cups Roma tomatoes, diced

1½ cups *heirloom tomatoes* (preferably of differing colors and sizes), diced

½ cup green bell pepper, diced

½ cup orange, yellow, or red bell pepper, diced

½ cup red onion, diced

2 jalapeño peppers, ribs and seeds removed, and finely diced

⅓ cup chopped fresh cilantro

¼ cup green onion, thinly sliced

2 TB. garlic, minced

Juice of 1 lime

1 tsp. sea salt

½ tsp. freshly ground black pepper or garlic pepper

1. In a large bowl, combine Roma tomatoes, heirloom tomatoes, green bell pepper, orange bell pepper, red onion, jalapeño peppers, cilantro, green onion, garlic, lime juice, sea salt, and pepper, and stir well. Cover and set aside for 30 minutes or more to allow flavors to blend.

2. Serve with tortilla chips or use as a sauce for beans, tacos, burritos, or other Mexican dishes. Store salsa in an airtight container in the refrigerator for up to 5 days.

Variation: To add even more color and flavor, add 1 cup cooked black beans or other beans of choice.

> **DEFINITION**
>
> **Heirloom tomatoes** are cultivated using seeds that have been passed down from generation to generation and are prized by growers and consumers for their exceptional flavor. They can be found in a wide variety of green, yellow, orange, pink, red, red-brown, purple-black, and even striped colors; in round, elongated, and bulging shapes of various sizes; and with flavors that range from sweet or savory to slightly bitter.

Roasted Tomatillo and Avocado Salsa

The addition of diced avocado provides some creamy texture, as well as a cooling effect, to this spicy, green-hued salsa.

Yield:	Prep time:	Cook time:	Serving size:
2 cups	5 to 7 minutes	10 to 12 minutes	¼ cup

4 to 6 *tomatillos,* husked and cut into quarters

⅔ cup yellow onion, diced

2 jalapeño peppers or 1 pasilla chile pepper, ribs and seeds removed, and finely diced

4 large garlic cloves

1 cup chopped fresh cilantro

¼ cup green onion, thinly sliced

Juice of 1 lime

¾ tsp. dried oregano

½ tsp. ground coriander

1 medium Hass avocado, peeled, pitted, and cut into ½-in. cubes

Sea salt

Freshly ground black pepper

1. Preheat the oven to 425°F. Line a large cookie sheet with parchment paper or a Silpat liner.

2. Place tomatillos, onion, and jalapeño peppers on the prepared cookie sheet. Bake for 8 to 10 minutes or until soft and lightly browned around the edges. Remove from the oven.

3. Transfer tomatillos, yellow onion, and jalapeño peppers to a blender or food processor fitted with an S blade. Add garlic, and process for 1 minute or until roughly chopped.

4. Add cilantro, green onion, lime juice, oregano, and coriander, and pulse several times or until as smooth or chunky as desired.

5. Transfer tomatillo mixture to a medium bowl, and stir in Hass avocado. Taste and season with sea salt and pepper as desired.

6. Serve as a sauce for cooked beans, burritos, tacos, enchiladas, or other Mexican dishes, or as a dip with tortilla chips. Store salsa in an airtight container in the refrigerator for up to 5 days.

Variation: For a milder-flavored salsa, place tomatillos, onion, and enough water to cover them, in a medium saucepan, and bring to a boil over high heat. Cover, reduce heat to low, and simmer for 10 to 12 minutes or until tomatillos are tender. Remove tomatillos and onion from the cooking liquid, and transfer to a blender or food processor. Add the remaining ingredients, except Hass avocado, and process as described.

DEFINITION

Tomatillos are small, round, pale-green fruits of the tomatillo plant that grow enclosed in a protective, paperlike husk. They're often mistaken for green, unripened tomatoes, but they differ greatly, and in comparison to their red tomato cousins, and have a tart flavor and much firmer texture. Look for tomatillos alongside tomatoes in your local grocery or natural foods store, or Latino specialty market.

Sauces Galore and More

Chapter

9

In This Chapter

- Oust the oil with our Oil Replacer
- Tomato- and veggie-based sauces
- Cornstarch-thickened creations
- Soy-based sour cream and mayo

Although store-bought sauces and condiments are convenient, there's no substitute for fresh. Fresh is best for achieving vibrant colors, crisp textures, and the fullest, most intense and robust flavor. Plus there's the bountiful health benefits of home-made. Forget additives and preservatives; you'll know precisely what went into your concoction and feel confident you're doing your body good.

To help you make healthier versions of your favorite toppers, we've developed an Oil Replacer made with cornstarch that can be used to replace all or part of the oil typically used to make sauces and salad dressings. And let's not forget cornstarch. This simple starch is affordable, readily available, and shines at thickening and binding together your gluten-free recipes.

The tasty toppings featured in this chapter can quickly turn humdrum or lackluster food into a taste sensation! We've offered a few suggestions with each recipe, but you're bound to find even more ways to use them. Best of all, most of these recipes can be stored for up to a week in the refrigerator. So you can invest minimal time creating them and enjoy them all week. You'll be saving money on the store-bought versions all while indulging your taste buds in fresh and fabulous flavor.

Oil Replacer

This oil substitute acts as a binder in revamping sauces and salad dressing recipes to replace all or part of the oil typically called for.

Yield:	Prep time:	Cook time:	Serving size:
2 cups	1 or 2 minutes	3 to 5 minutes	2 to 4 tablespoons

2 cups water

2 TB. cornstarch

¾ tsp. xanthan gum

1. In a small saucepan, whisk together water, cornstarch, and xanthan gum, and cook over medium heat, whisking often, for 3 to 5 minutes or until thickened. Remove from heat, and set aside to cool.

2. Transfer mixture to an airtight container. Store oil replacer in the refrigerator for up to 2 weeks.

MEATLESS AND WHEATLESS

To make a more flavorful oil replacer, replace the water with low-sodium vegetable broth. If you're making a fruit-flavored dressing, use apple juice or another variety of fruit juice that will complement the flavor of your salad dressing.

Five-Minute Marinara

Fire-roasted crushed tomatoes and a little red wine give this sauce an authentic Italian flavor without olive oil. We've dramatically decreased the cooking time by preparing it in a large skillet rather than a pot.

Yield:	Prep time:	Cook time:	Serving size:
3½ cups	2 or 3 minutes	5 minutes	½ cup

⅓ cup white or yellow onion, finely diced

3 TB. low-sodium vegetable broth or water

1½ TB. garlic, minced

1 tsp. dried basil

1 tsp. dried oregano

½ tsp. sea salt

¼ tsp. freshly ground black pepper

¼ tsp. crushed red pepper flakes

1 (28-oz.) can fire-roasted crushed tomatoes

2 TB. red wine

1. Place a large, nonstick skillet over medium-high heat. Add white onion and vegetable broth, and cook, stirring often, for 1 minute.

2. Add garlic, basil, oregano, sea salt, pepper, and crushed red pepper flakes, and cook, stirring often, for 1 more minute.

3. Stir in crushed tomatoes and red wine, reduce heat to low, and simmer for 3 minutes to blend flavors. Remove from heat.

4. Use as a sauce for pizza, gluten-free pasta, or other dishes, as well as on sandwiches. Store sauce in an airtight container in the refrigerator for up to 5 days.

Variation: For a nonalcoholic marinara sauce, feel free to omit the red wine. For an even more flavorful sauce, replace the dried basil with ¼ cup chopped fresh basil. To turn this into **Vodka Tomato Sauce,** add ½ cup soy milk or other nondairy milk, ¼ cup vodka, and 1 tablespoon Spicy Sprinkles or Italian Herb Sprinkles (recipe and variation in Chapter 6) to the finished marinara sauce, and simmer for 2 more minutes.

MEATLESS AND WHEATLESS

We often call for fire-roasted tomato products in this book because they have a far superior flavor to other varieties of canned tomatoes products. We like the ones made by Muir Glen using organic tomatoes that have been roasted over an open fire.

Bourbon Blues BBQ Sauce

Use this smoky, spicy, bourbon-spiked sauce on sandwiches or wraps, on pieces of tofu or tempeh, or in a batch of baked beans.

Yield:	Prep time:	Serving size:
2 cups	3 to 5 minutes	¼ cup

½ cup tomato paste

½ cup apple cider vinegar

¼ cup maple syrup, or 2 TB. maple syrup and 2 TB. sorghum syrup

¼ cup bourbon whiskey

¼ cup red onion, finely diced

2½ TB. wheat-free tamari

2 TB. garlic, minced

1 TB. fresh ginger, minced

1 TB. spicy brown mustard

¼ tsp. cayenne or chipotle chili powder

¼ tsp. smoked paprika

¼ tsp. smoked sea salt

¼ tsp. freshly ground black pepper or garlic pepper

1. In a blender or food processor fitted with an S blade, combine tomato paste, apple cider vinegar, maple syrup, bourbon, red onion, tamari, garlic, ginger, brown mustard, cayenne, smoked paprika, smoked sea salt, and pepper, and process for 1 or 2 minutes or until smooth. Scrape down the sides of the container with a spatula, and process for 15 more seconds.

2. Store sauce in an airtight container in the refrigerator for up to 2 weeks.

Variation: For a nonalcoholic BBQ sauce, omit the bourbon. For an even hotter BBQ sauce, add 1 diced jalapeño pepper.

CORNUCOPIA

Most experts agree that gluten doesn't survive the distillation process, but it's best to check with the manufacturer of your favorite distilled spirit to verify if it's both vegan and gluten free. That being said, both Kentucky and Tennessee are known for making great bourbon whiskey, so you can decide for yourself what type of bourbon whiskey you use in this recipe. Our favorite Kentucky bourbon whiskey is Maker's Mark, and from Tennessee, it's Jack Daniel's, naturally.

Miso-Peanut Sauce

A generous amount of *miso*, lime juice, and fresh garlic and ginger give this peanut butter–based sauce a nice, tangy flavor.

Yield:	Prep time:	Serving size:
¾ cup	2 or 3 minutes	2 tablespoons

⅓ cup natural peanut butter

⅓ cup low-sodium vegetable broth or water

2 TB. mellow miso or other miso

Juice of 1 lime

1½ TB. wheat-free tamari

2 tsp. garlic, minced

2 tsp. fresh ginger, minced

1½ tsp. toasted sesame oil

¼ tsp. freshly ground black pepper or garlic pepper

⅛ tsp. crushed red pepper flakes or cayenne

1. In a blender or food processor fitted with an S blade, combine peanut butter, vegetable broth, and mellow miso, and process for 30 seconds. Scrape down the sides of the container with a spatula.

2. Add lime juice, tamari, garlic, ginger, toasted sesame oil, pepper, and crushed red pepper flakes, and process for 1 or 2 minutes or until smooth.

3. Use as a sauce or accompaniment for sandwiches, wraps, or nori rolls, or as a dressing for salads, fresh or cooked vegetables, grains, gluten-free noodles, stir-fries, or other main or side dishes. Store sauce in an airtight container in the refrigerator for up to 5 to 7 days.

Variation: Feel free to replace the peanut butter with other nut or seed butters, such as cashew, almond, sunflower, or soy nut butter.

Plant-Based Dietitian Recommends: Omit the oil.

DEFINITION

Miso is a thick paste made from fermenting soybeans with a little salt and koji, which is made by inoculating grains (typically rice) with a beneficial type of mold. It has a very unique flavor, which is somewhat salty, sweet, and savory all at the same time, and is available in several varieties. Be sure to carefully check the ingredients list because some varieties contain barley and are not gluten free.

Béchamel Sauce

Cornstarch works its magic at thickening this lightly seasoned revamp of the classic Béchamel sauce (a.k.a. white sauce), and you'll be pleased to know it's oil free, too.

Yield:	Prep time:	Cook time:	Serving size:
2 cups	1 or 2 minutes	3 to 5 minutes	¼ cup

2½ TB. cornstarch

1 TB. nutritional yeast flakes

1 tsp. onion powder

1 tsp. garlic powder or garlic granules

½ tsp. sea salt

¼ tsp. freshly ground black pepper or garlic pepper

¼ tsp. freshly grated nutmeg

2 cups soy milk or other nondairy milk

1. In a small saucepan, combine cornstarch, nutritional yeast flakes, onion powder, garlic powder, sea salt, pepper, and nutmeg, and whisk well. Whisk in soy milk, and cook over medium heat, whisking often, for 3 to 5 minutes or until thickened. Remove from heat.

2. Use as a sauce over vegetables, in stews or casseroles, or in main dishes. Serve hot. Store sauce in an airtight container in the refrigerator for up to 1 week.

Variation: For a more flavorful **Lite White Sauce,** replace 1 cup soy milk with 1 cup low-sodium vegetable broth, or if you prefer, use ¾ cup vegetable broth and ¼ cup white wine.

CORNUCOPIA

Knowing how to make a basic Béchamel sauce can be quite useful to the home cook. You can use this versatile sauce as a base for casseroles and creamy soups, to top your favorite pasta and vegetable dishes, or with a few simple additions, to make other sauces.

Roasted Onion and Garlic Gravy

Roasting the onion and garlic adds a lot to the savory flavor of this tasty gravy.

Yield:	Prep time:	Cook time:	Serving size:
2½ cups	5 to 7 minutes	25 to 30 minutes	¼ cup

½ cup white or yellow onion, cut into 1-in.-wide slices

6 large garlic cloves

2 cups low-sodium vegetable broth or water

3 TB. nutritional yeast flakes

2 TB. cornstarch

1 TB. wheat-free tamari

1 TB. chopped fresh thyme or 1 tsp. dried thyme

½ tsp. sea salt

¼ tsp. freshly ground black pepper or garlic pepper

1. Preheat the oven to 375°F.

2. Cut a 6-inch-square piece of parchment paper, and place it on top of an 8×12-inch piece of aluminum foil. Place white onion and garlic in the center of the parchment paper, and fold over the edges of the paper to enclose them. Gather the corners of the aluminum foil, crimp to enclose the parchment paper, and place it in a pie pan.

3. Bake for 15 to 20 minutes or until white onion and garlic in the packet feel soft when gently squeezed. Remove from the oven and let cool for 5 minutes.

4. Transfer white onion and garlic to a blender or food processor fitted with an S blade. Add 1 cup vegetable broth, and process for 1 or 2 minutes or until smooth. Scrape down the sides of the container with a spatula, and process for 15 more seconds.

5. Add remaining 1 cup vegetable broth, nutritional yeast flakes, cornstarch, tamari, thyme, sea salt, and pepper, and process for 1 more minute.

6. Transfer mixture to a medium saucepan, and cook over medium heat, whisking often, for 3 or 4 minutes or until thickened. Remove from heat.

7. Serve gravy over mashed potatoes, biscuits, grains, vegetables, and other side dishes, or use as a sauce in casseroles. Store gravy in an airtight container in the refrigerator for up to 1 week or in the freezer for up to 3 months.

Variation: For added flavor, replace $\frac{1}{2}$ cup vegetable broth with white wine. For corn-free gravy, replace the cornstarch with chickpea/garbanzo bean flour. To make **Country-Style Onion Gravy,** instead of roasting them, chop the white onion and garlic, and place them in a medium saucepan. Add $\frac{1}{3}$ cup vegetable broth, and cook over medium heat, stirring often, for 5 minutes or until soft. In a small bowl, whisk together remaining $1\frac{2}{3}$ cups vegetable broth and other ingredients, add it to onion mixture, and cook, whisking often, for 3 or 4 more minutes or until thickened.

MEATLESS AND WHEATLESS

Fresh herbs are typically sold in small bunches, and you often only need a small amount when making a recipe, rather than the whole bunch. But don't stress over how to not let the extra thyme go to waste. You can chop it all, place it in an airtight container or zipper-lock bag, and freeze it for later use. You can also do this with rosemary, tarragon, oregano, marjoram, and chives.

Basil, Spinach, and Pumpkin Seed Pesto

In this remake of classic Genovese pesto, pumpkin seeds add a nutty flavor and texture, fresh basil pairs with baby spinach, and miso and nutritional yeast flakes provide a bit of saltiness and cheesy flavor.

Yield:	Prep time:	Serving size:
$1\frac{1}{2}$ cups	5 minutes	2 tablespoons

$\frac{1}{3}$ cup raw pumpkin seeds

$1\frac{1}{2}$ cups fresh basil leaves, tightly packed

$1\frac{1}{2}$ cups baby spinach, tightly packed

4 large garlic cloves

$\frac{1}{2}$ cup Oil Replacer (recipe earlier in this chapter)

2 TB. mellow miso

2 TB. nutritional yeast flakes, Spicy Sprinkles (recipe in Chapter 6), or Italian Herb Sprinkles (variation in Chapter 6)

$\frac{1}{4}$ tsp. sea salt

$\frac{1}{4}$ tsp. freshly ground black pepper or garlic pepper

$\frac{1}{4}$ tsp. crushed red pepper flakes

1. In a food processor fitted with an S blade, place pumpkin seeds, and process for 1 minute or until finely ground. Add basil, spinach, and garlic, and process for 1 minute or until roughly chopped. Scrape down the sides of the container with a spatula.

2. Add Oil Replacer, mellow miso, nutritional yeast flakes, sea salt, pepper, and crushed red pepper flakes, and process for 1 or 2 more minutes or until a smooth paste forms.

3. Use to flavor gluten-free pasta, grains, vegetable dishes, soups, and sauces, or use as a spread for wraps, sandwiches, or on slices of bread. Store pesto in an airtight container in the refrigerator for up to 5 to 7 days, or in the freezer for up to 3 months.

Variation: Feel free to replace the pumpkin seeds with hemp seeds, walnuts, pistachios, or other seeds or nuts, or substitute Italian flat-leaf parsley for the spinach. For a pesto with a little bite to it, replace the spinach with arugula.

MEATLESS AND WHEATLESS

Pesto is such a versatile condiment and a great go-to ingredient for flavoring your favorite dishes, we've come up with a technique so you can have it on hand: mound 2 tablespoons pesto on a parchment paper–lined cookie sheet, and freeze until solid. Transfer the pesto mounds to an airtight container or zipper-lock bag, label and date it, and keep it in the freezer for pesto anytime.

Tofu Sour Cream

Within minutes, you can make your own light, creamy, and slightly tangy mock sour cream simply by blending together some *silken tofu* with lemon juice and a few other ingredients.

Yield:	Prep time:	Serving size:
2½ cups	2 or 3 minutes, plus 30 minutes chill time	2 tablespoons

1 (12-oz.) pkg. firm or extra-firm silken tofu

¼ cup soy milk or other nondairy milk

3 TB. lemon juice

1 TB. nutritional yeast flakes

1 TB. gluten-free brown rice syrup

½ tsp. sea salt

1. Using your fingers, crumble tofu into a blender or food processor fitted with an S blade. Add soy milk, lemon juice, nutritional yeast flakes, brown rice syrup, and sea salt, and process for 1 minute. Scrape down the sides of the container with a spatula, and process for 1 more minute or until smooth.

2. Transfer mixture to an airtight container, and chill for 30 minutes or more to allow flavors to blend.

3. Serve as a topping for baked potatoes, soups, salads, and other dishes as desired. Store sour cream in an airtight container in the refrigerator for up to 1 week.

Variation: You can change the flavor of the sour cream by adding 2 or more tablespoons chopped fresh herbs such as basil, dill, cilantro, parsley, or mint.

DEFINITION

Silken tofu is made from soybeans and has a creamy, velvety-smooth texture. The process for making silken tofu differs slightly from regular tofu in that the soy milk curds and excess water aren't separated during production. Depending on the silken tofu's final texture, it's labeled soft, firm, or extra-firm. Silken tofu is often blended for making sauces, salad dressings, beverages, desserts, and baked goods.

Reduced-Fat Soy Milk Mayo

Store-bought vegan mayonnaise is typically made with a generous amount of oil. This soy milk–based recipe contains only a few tablespoons of olive oil yet has a creamy texture and mouthfeel similar to its high-fat counterparts.

Yield:	Prep time:	Serving size:
2 cups	8 to 10 minutes	1 tablespoon

²/₃ cup water	1¹/₂ tsp. nutritional yeast flakes
¹/₄ cup cornstarch	1¹/₂ tsp. sea salt
2 tsp. agar powder or 2 TB. agar-agar flakes	1 tsp. onion powder
1 cup soy milk or other nondairy milk	¹/₂ tsp. garlic powder or garlic granules
2 tsp. Dijon mustard	¹/₄ cup olive oil
2 tsp. gluten-free brown rice syrup	1 TB. apple cider vinegar
	1 TB. lemon juice

1. In a small saucepan, combine water, cornstarch, and agar powder, and cook over high heat, whisking often, for 3 to 5 minutes or until thickened. Remove from heat.

2. Meanwhile, in a blender, combine soy milk, Dijon mustard, brown rice syrup, nutritional yeast flakes, sea salt, onion powder, and garlic powder, and blend for 30 seconds. Add cornstarch mixture, and blend for 30 seconds. Scrape down the sides of the container with a spatula.

3. With the blender running, through the feed tube (or remove the lid), slowly add olive oil, followed by apple cider vinegar and lemon juice, and process for 1 more minute.

4. Transfer mayo to an airtight container and chill for 1 hour or more to allow flavors to blend, and for mayo to thicken slightly.

5. Use as a condiment on sandwiches or wraps, as an ingredient in salad dressings or dips, and in your other favorite recipes. Store mayo in the refrigerator for up to 2 weeks.

Variation: You can adapt this recipe to make flavored mayonnaise by adding additional ingredients such as sun-dried tomatoes; chipotle chili powder; curry powder; wasabi powder; or chopped fresh basil, dill, parsley, or other herbs.

Plant-Based Dietitian Recommends: Opt for this oil-free variation of mayonnaise: in a blender, combine 1 (12-ounce) package firm or extra-firm silken tofu, $1\frac{1}{2}$ tablespoons lemon juice, 1 teaspoon brown rice syrup, 1 teaspoon Dijon mustard, $\frac{1}{2}$ teaspoon sea salt, $\frac{1}{2}$ teaspoon onion powder, and $\frac{1}{4}$ teaspoon garlic powder, and blend for 1 or 2 minutes or until smooth and creamy.

CORNUCOPIA

You may be wondering what the difference is between garlic powder and garlic granules. They have similar flavor, but the major difference is texture or size. Garlic powder is much finer than garlic granules. Also, garlic powder dissolves almost instantly when incorporated into any dish, in comparison to garlic granules, which often take a few minutes to fully combine and release their flavor.

Ready for Lunch?

Whether you're going to be brown-bagging it, having your girlfriends (or boyfriends) over for a sit-down luncheon, or simply in need of something hearty to wrap your hands around on a lazy afternoon, Part 4 provides plenty of ideas for filling midday meals.

No matter what your appetite or need may be, you're bound to find something to appeal to your tastes in Part 4. For those who prefer to eat light or all-raw until dinner, we included a whole chapter that features both leafy and veggie-packed salads.

We've also amassed quite a selection of homemade and gluten-free meatless meats, and filling sandwiches of all sorts that utilize many of them, as well as the other bread, buns, condiments, and flavorful add-ins found throughout this book.

And for those who enjoy a good cup or bowlful of soul-satisfying soup, either alone, with a bit of bread, or in a combo with salad or sandwich, you're bound to find one or more of the soups in this part to your liking.

Satisfying Salads

In This Chapter

- DIY sprouts
- All-raw salads and slaws
- Palate-pleasing potato and pasta salads

For those of you who don't get enough raw veggies as a part of your daily diet, the Plant-Based Dietitian (Julieanna) and the Vegan Chef (Beverly) are here to help! We both love eating leafy greens, crunchy crucifers, earthy roots, and tons of other fresh, frozen, and canned veggies, as well as fruits, and beans and other legumes as a part of our salad-based meals. So in this chapter, we've include a handful of our favorite salads and slaws we hope will inspire you to follow in our produce-eating footsteps.

For those with simple tastes, try drizzling a little apple cider vinegar or lemon juice on your salad, rather than using a prepared salad dressing. Of course, it's quite easy to mix up a batch of your own homemade salad dressing, but if you want to go the store-bought bottled route, really scrutinize the ingredients and nutritional information so you can make the wisest choices for topping your salad bowl.

Also, there's no need to drown your salads in dressing. Go light on the dressing at first, give it a taste, and if you think it needs a little more, just drizzle a bit more over the top. Remember, you can always add, but you can't take away.

Things Are Sprouting Up All Over

Sprouts are real superfoods. During the process of sprouting, many significant changes occur in the seed that benefit the consumer. Antinutrients, those that inhibit absorption of important vitamins and minerals, are disabled. Stored nutrients in the seed are released. Vitamins, minerals, phytonutrients, enzymes, and essential fatty acids multiply and become more easily digestible. Sprouts are also excellent sources of fiber and high-quality protein.

Humble sprouts can add enormous flavor and texture to your salads, sandwiches, and wraps, as well as your favorite grain, noodle, and other dishes. Each type of sprout has its own distinct flavor, from mild red lentil and sweet clover to spicy radish and perfumed fenugreek.

MEATLESS AND WHEATLESS

You can find sprouting seeds in packages and bulk bins of most natural foods stores, or check online.

The following table offers a breakdown by variety of how much sprouting seeds you need, how many days they take to sprout, and their yield.

Seed	How Much You Need	Days to Sprout	Yield
Alfalfa	3 tablespoons	3 to 5 days	approximately 3 or 4 cups
Broccoli	2 tablespoons	3 to 5 days	2 cups
Clover and red clover	3 tablespoons	4 to 6 days	approximately 3 or 4 cups
Fenugreek	$\frac{1}{4}$ cup	4 to 6 days	3 cups
Mung bean	$\frac{1}{3}$ cup	4 to 6 days	4 cups
Radish	3 tablespoons	3 to 5 days	3 or 4 cups
Red lentil	$\frac{1}{2}$ cup	3 or 4 days	3 or 4 cups

We find that the water method, rather than growing them in soil, is much easier for growing sprouts on a small scale. All you need to start your own sprout garden are some sprouting jars with assorted screen lids, or quart-sized canning jars with metal rings and some fine mesh round screens. Both of these options are available through online sources or in most natural foods, kitchen supply, or hardware stores.

Check out the Fresh and Flavorful Sprouts recipe in this chapter for further sprouting instructions and tips.

The Dirty Dozen and the Clean 15

We encourage everyone to eat as much organically grown produce as possible because the use of harmful pesticides, herbicides, and fungicides is rampant in conventionally grown produce. In fact, some produce varieties, when tested for these contaminants, were found to contain from 47 to 67 different chemicals, and some varieties of apples contained over 90! Also, contrary to myth, you cannot remove these residues by simply washing your produce with running water. That only removes dirt and other such debris, and residues can still be found in the internal flesh of the produce. Produce that has tough or firm outer skins, such as pineapples or corn, tend to soak up fewer pesticides than soft-skinned produce, like berries and stone fruits.

However, it's much more important for you to consume plenty of fruits and vegetables than to avoid them due to inability to find or afford organically grown options. We recommend prioritizing organic produce first, followed by conventionally grown, because eating an abundance of fruits and veggies every day is one of the best habits you can get into for optimal health and disease prevention.

To help you prioritize when to opt for organic over conventionally grown produce, the Environmental Working Group created two handy lists of items with the most pesticides and those with the least. The "Dirty Dozen" list includes celery, peaches, strawberries, apples, blueberries, nectarines, bell peppers, spinach, kale, cherries, potatoes, and grapes. We advise you to buy these organic.

The "Clean 15" were found to contain fewer traces of pesticides and, therefore, are safer to consume in nonorganic form. Onions, avocados, sweet corn, pineapples, mangoes, sweet peas, asparagus, kiwi, cabbage, eggplant, cantaloupe, watermelon, grapefruit, sweet potatoes, and honeydew melon are all on this list.

Fresh and Flavorful Sprouts

Ready to grow some sprouts? Grab your seeds, sprouting jars, and lids, and let's get started. After a few days of diligent rinsing and draining, you'll be feasting on some of the finest-tasting sprouts around.

Yield:	Prep time:	Serving size:
2 to 4 cups, depending on variety	6 hours soak time, plus 3 to 7 days growing time	$\frac{1}{4}$ to $\frac{1}{2}$ cup

3 TB. to $\frac{1}{2}$ cup sprouting seeds of choice	Water

1. Place sprouting seeds in a sprouting jar, cover with 3 inches water, secure mesh screen and/or lid on jar, and leave to soak for 6 hours or overnight. Drain off and discard soaking water.

2. To rinse sprouts, fill jar with enough water to cover seeds, drain off water, and repeat the procedure two more times.

3. Invert the jar at an angle in a small bowl, and set aside to drain away from direct sunlight or overhead lighting. Repeat rinse and draining procedure two more times throughout the day.

4. Continue the rinsing and draining procedure for the next few days until seeds begin to have small green leaves and several-inch-long stems. When the sprouts start to leaf out, they're ready to harvest. Transfer the sprouts to an airtight container, and use immediately or store in the refrigerator for up to 3 days.

Variation: To add variety to your meals, top them with 1 or more types of sprouts.

MEATLESS AND WHEATLESS

You can buy many varieties of ready-to-eat fresh sprouts at grocery and natural foods stores. Try alfalfa or radish sprouts, for example. However, you should know that in the last few years, sprouts have been recalled due to contamination concerns. But don't let this stop you from enjoying these tender seedlings because it's quite easy to start your own countertop sprout garden.

Fresh Fruit, Avocado, and Spinach Salad

This fresh and fruity salad features sweet and juicy mango, pineapple, kiwi, and red bell peppers with creamy chunks of avocado.

Yield:	Prep time:	Serving size:
6 cups	10 to 15 minutes	1½ cups

½ cup mango, peeled, pitted, and diced

½ cup pineapple tidbits or chunks

⅓ cup red bell pepper, diced

1 kiwi, peeled, cut into quarters lengthwise, and sliced

¼ cup red onion, diced

2 TB. jalapeño pepper, ribs and seeds removed, and finely diced

2 TB. chopped fresh cilantro

1 medium Hass avocado, peeled, pitted, and diced

1 TB. lime juice

Sea salt

Freshly ground black pepper

4 cups baby spinach, tightly packed

¼ cup sliced raw almonds

Salad dressing of choice (preferably a fruit-based one)

1. In a medium bowl, combine mango, pineapple, red bell pepper, kiwi, red onion, jalapeño pepper, and cilantro, and stir well.

2. Add Hass avocado, drizzle lime juice directly over top, and stir gently to combine. Taste and season with sea salt and pepper as desired.

3. Evenly divide spinach among 4 plates. For each serving, place ½ cup fruit mixture on top of spinach, and sprinkle 1 tablespoon sliced almonds over top. Drizzle a little of your favorite salad dressing over each portion, and serve.

Variation: For added flavor and texture, top individual servings with ¼ cup or more Fresh and Flavorful Sprouts using red clover or fenugreek (recipe earlier in chapter). Feel free to replace the baby spinach with arugula or mixed baby greens.

MEATLESS AND WHEATLESS

Buying bags of prewashed greens helps you easily incorporate more leafy greens in your daily diet and can save you a lot of time when making fresh salads and cooked dishes. Check the produce section and you're sure to find several bagged leafy greens options. Some brands also have chopped cabbages, carrots, and other ingredients added.

Orchard Medley and Mixed Greens Salad

We suggest choosing baby mixed greens for this fruit and nut mixed greens salad. They contain a lot of red-colored greens to complement the colors of the crisp pears and apple, dried cranberries, and pomegranate seeds.

Yield:	Prep time:	Serving size:
9 cups	10 to 15 minutes	1½ cups

2 large Anjou pears or other pears, cored and thinly sliced

1 large Gala or Fuji apple, cored and thinly sliced

1 TB. lemon juice

1 (5-oz.) pkg. mixed greens of choice

½ cup dried cranberries or dried cherries

½ cup toasted pecans, roughly chopped

½ cup toasted hazelnuts or walnuts, roughly chopped

Seeds of 1 large pomegranate

Salad dressing of choice (preferably a vinaigrette or fruit-based one)

1. In a medium bowl, combine pears and apple, drizzle lemon juice over top, and gently toss to evenly coat.

2. In a large bowl, combine mixed greens, pear-apple mixture, dried cranberries, pecans, and hazelnuts, and toss gently to combine. Sprinkle pomegranate seeds over top of salad, and serve. Drizzle salad dressing over entire salad and toss, or simply drizzle dressings over individual servings as desired.

Variation: You can substitute Asian pears and other varieties of apples in this salad, as well as substitute other varieties of dried fruits, such as raisins, currants, or chopped dates or apricots. You can also replace one or more of the nuts with sunflower or pumpkin seeds.

AGAINST THE GRAIN

Many dried fruit manufacturers often use sulfites, such as sulfur dioxide, to help preserve the vibrant color of their dried fruits. These preservatives can cause allergic and sometimes life-threatening reactions, such as hives or skin rashes, migraines, swelling of the throat, and difficulty breathing. Fortunately, the FDA requires all packaged foods that contain sulfites to clearly state so on their product labels.

Corn, Squash, and Cherry Tomato Salad

Make this simple and refreshing Mexican-inspired salad during the summer when local farmers' markets, grocery stores, or even your own garden are overflowing with fresh corn, squashes, and ripe and juicy cherry tomatoes.

Yield:	Prep time:	Serving size:
5 cups	5 to 7 minutes	1 cup

2 cups fresh or frozen cut corn kernels

1½ cups pear, grape, or cherry tomatoes, cut in ½ (preferably of differing colors)

⅔ cup yellow summer squash, cut in ½ lengthwise and thinly sliced

⅔ cup zucchini, cut in ½ lengthwise and thinly sliced

¼ cup green onion, thinly sliced

¼ cup raw pumpkin seeds

¼ cup chopped fresh cilantro or basil

2 TB. chopped fresh parsley

1½ TB. olive oil

1 TB. red wine vinegar

1 TB. garlic, minced

1 tsp. chili powder

½ tsp. ground cumin

Sea salt

Freshly ground black pepper

1. In a medium bowl, combine corn, pear tomatoes, yellow summer squash, zucchini, green onion, pumpkin seeds, cilantro, and parsley.

2. In a small bowl, whisk together olive oil, red wine vinegar, garlic, chili powder, and cumin.

3. Pour dressing over corn mixture, and stir well to combine. Taste and season with sea salt and pepper as desired. Set aside for 15 minutes to allow flavors to blend. Serve at room temperature.

Variation: For added color and texture, add 1 cup canned red or black beans. You also can toss this salad with cooked gluten-free pasta for a quick and easy pasta salad or main dish.

Plant-Based Dietitian Recommends: Omit the oil.

Marinated Red Potato Salad

This good-for-you potato salad contains less than 1 tablespoon oil in the entire salad, yet has a fantastic flavor thanks to the robust red wine vinegar, fresh herbs, and crisp vegetables.

Yield:	Prep time:	Cook time:	Serving size:
7 to 8 cups	15 minutes	8 to 10 minutes	1 cup

3 lb. red-skinned potatoes (about 6 or 7 large potatoes), cut into quarters lengthwise and thinly sliced

1 cup celery, cut in $\frac{1}{2}$ lengthwise and thinly sliced

$\frac{1}{2}$ cup red onion, finely diced

$\frac{1}{2}$ cup green onion, thinly sliced

$\frac{1}{4}$ cup chopped fresh parsley

2 TB. chopped fresh dill or 2 tsp. dried dill weed

$\frac{1}{4}$ cup low-sodium vegetable broth

$\frac{1}{4}$ cup red wine vinegar

3 TB. Oil Replacer (recipe in Chapter 9)

2 TB. nutritional yeast flakes

2 tsp. olive oil

$\frac{3}{4}$ tsp. sea salt

$\frac{1}{2}$ tsp. freshly ground black pepper or garlic pepper

1. In a large pot, place red-skinned potatoes, cover with water, and cook over medium heat for 8 to 10 minutes or until potatoes are just tender and can be easily pierced with a knife. Drain potatoes in a colander, rinse with cold water, and drain well again.

2. Transfer potatoes to a large bowl. Add celery, red onion, green onion, parsley, and dill, and stir gently to combine.

3. In a small bowl, whisk together vegetable broth, red wine vinegar, Oil Replacer, nutritional yeast flakes, olive oil, sea salt, and pepper.

4. Pour dressing over potato mixture, and stir gently until evenly coated. Serve immediately, or set aside for 15 minutes or more to allow flavors to blend.

Variation: Feel free to replace the red-skinned potatoes with Yukon gold potatoes, purple potatoes, or fingerling potatoes. You can create a **Dijonnaise Potato Salad** by replacing the vegetable broth and Oil Replacer with 6 tablespoons Reduced-Fat Soy Milk Mayo (recipe in Chapter 9) and 3 tablespoons Dijon mustard.

Plant-Based Dietitian Recommends: Omit the oil or add an additional 1 tablespoon Oil Replacer.

CORNUCOPIA

The potato originated in Peru, and amazingly, more than half of the thousands of potato varieties available worldwide are still found there and throughout the Andes Mountain region. These tasty spuds are serious business in the global economy. In fact, potatoes are the world's fourth-largest food crop but continue to give the top three—rice, wheat, and corn—a run for their money.

Southwestern Sweet Potato Salad

In the Southwestern United States, beans, corn, bell peppers, jalapeños, and a generous amount of spices are a favorite combination. These treasured ingredients are combined with tender sweet potatoes in this colorful and crunchy salad.

Yield:	Prep time:	Cook time:	Serving size:
8 cups	15 to 20 minutes	8 to 10 minutes	1 cup

2 large sweet potatoes or garnet yams, peeled, cut into quarters lengthwise, and thinly sliced

1 (15-oz.) can black beans or black soybeans, drained and rinsed

1 cup green bell pepper, diced

1 cup red bell pepper, diced

$\frac{1}{2}$ cup fresh or frozen cut corn kernels

$\frac{1}{4}$ cup green onion, thinly sliced

1 jalapeño pepper, ribs and seeds removed, and finely diced

$\frac{1}{4}$ cup chopped fresh cilantro

$\frac{1}{4}$ cup chopped fresh parsley

$\frac{1}{4}$ cup raw pumpkin seeds

2 TB. olive oil

2 TB. apple cider vinegar

Juice of 1 lime

4 tsp. garlic, minced

1 tsp. dried oregano

1 tsp. chili powder

$\frac{3}{4}$ tsp. ground cumin

$\frac{1}{2}$ tsp. ground coriander

$\frac{1}{2}$ tsp. sea salt

$\frac{1}{4}$ tsp. freshly ground black pepper

1. In a large pot, place sweet potatoes, cover with water, and cook over medium heat for 8 to 10 minutes or until just tender and sweet potatoes can be pierced easily with a knife. Drain sweet potatoes in a colander, rinse with cold water, and drain well again.

2. Transfer sweet potatoes to a large bowl. Add black beans, green bell pepper, red bell pepper, corn, green onion, jalapeño pepper, cilantro, parsley, and pumpkin seeds, and toss gently to combine.

3. In a small bowl, whisk together olive oil, apple cider vinegar, lime juice, garlic, oregano, chili powder, cumin, coriander, sea salt, and pepper.

4. Pour dressing over salad mixture, and stir gently until evenly coated. Serve immediately or set aside for 15 minutes or more to allow flavors to blend.

Variation: You can replace the black beans with red beans, kidney beans, or pinto beans, or if you're so inclined, use a combination of beans. Feel free to also add $\frac{1}{2}$ cup chopped zucchini or yellow summer squash or 1 diced Hass avocado for extra flavor and color. This salad is delicious served with tortilla chips and also makes a tasty filling for burritos or tacos.

Plant-Based Dietitian Recommends: Substitute 2 tablespoons vegetable broth or Oil Replacer for the oil.

> **CORNUCOPIA**
>
> Sweet potatoes are rich in carotenoids (provitamin A antioxidants), vitamins B_6 and C, as well as manganese, potassium, iron, and dietary fiber. Opt for the dark orange sweet potato varieties for the highest levels of vitamin A.

Pisano Pasta Salad

Transport your taste buds to the Italian countryside with one bite of this zesty pasta salad, made with plump cannellini beans, sun-dried tomatoes, artichokes, salty black olives, and fresh basil, all highlighted with an Italian dressing.

Yield:	Prep time:	Cook time:	Serving size:
6 or 7 cups	10 to 15 minutes	8 to 18 minutes (depending on pasta variety)	1 cup

1 (8-oz.) pkg. gluten-free fusilli, spirals, or other shaped pasta

⅔ cup store-bought Italian salad dressing or other salad dressing of choice

1½ TB. Spicy Sprinkles (recipe in Chapter 6) or Italian Herb Sprinkles (variation in Chapter 6), or nutritional yeast flakes

½ tsp. crushed red pepper flakes (optional)

¼ tsp. sea salt

¼ tsp. freshly ground black pepper

¾ cup canned cannellini beans or chickpeas, drained and rinsed

¾ cup zucchini, cut into quarters lengthwise and thinly sliced

½ cup artichoke hearts (packed in brine, not oil), roughly chopped

⅓ cup sun-dried tomato pieces

⅓ cup kalamata olives or other black olives, pitted and roughly chopped

⅓ cup chopped fresh basil

¼ cup toasted pine nuts (optional)

1. Fill a large saucepan ⅔ full of water, and bring to a boil over medium-high heat. Add fusilli, and cook, stirring often, according to package directions or until *al dente*. Drain pasta in a colander, rinse with cold water, and drain well again.

2. Transfer pasta to a large bowl. Add Italian salad dressing, Spicy Sprinkles, crushed red pepper flakes (if using), sea salt, and pepper, and stir gently until evenly coated.

3. Add cannellini beans, zucchini, artichoke hearts, sun-dried tomato pieces, kalamata olives, basil, and pine nuts (if using), and toss gently to combine. Set aside for 15 minutes or more to allow flavors to blend. Serve at room temperature.

Variation: To turn this salad into a one-plate meal, place individual servings on top of baby spinach or mixed baby greens. For a flavorful **Pesto Pasta Salad,** reserve $\frac{1}{2}$ cup of the pasta cooking water, mix it with $\frac{1}{2}$ cup Basil, Spinach, and Pumpkin Seed Pesto (recipe in Chapter 9), and use this mixture in place of the store-bought salad dressing.

DEFINITION

Al dente is an Italian phrase that literally means "to the tooth" or "to the bite." It's used to describe the proper degree of doneness when cooking pasta or other foods such as grains, beans, or vegetables. Al dente foods should be just tender, but still slightly firm and chewy when bitten into. If they're soft or mushy, they're overcooked.

Rainbow Vegetable Slaw

When it comes to nutrition, we encourage you to eat all the colors of the rainbow, and this crunchy vegetable slaw made with a wide assortment of leafy greens and earthy root vegetables can help do just that.

Yield:	Prep time:	Serving size:
9 cups	10 to 15 minutes	1½ cups

3 large leaves purple kale, roughly chopped

2 large leaves rainbow Swiss chard, roughly chopped

1 cup green cabbage, shredded

1 cup red cabbage, shredded

¾ cup carrots, shredded

¾ cup golden beets, peeled and shredded

¾ cup *watermelon daikon radish,* peeled and shredded

2 green onions, thinly sliced

1 stalk celery, diced

¼ cup chopped fresh cilantro

¼ cup chopped fresh parsley

Salad dressing of choice (preferably a vinaigrette or tahini-based one)

1. In a large bowl, combine purple kale, rainbow Swiss chard, green cabbage, red cabbage, carrots, golden beets, watermelon daikon radish, green onion, celery, cilantro, and parsley, and gently toss.

2. Drizzle ⅓ to ½ cup salad dressing as desired over slaw and toss gently until evenly coated, or drizzle dressing over individual servings as desired.

Variation: If you can't find golden beets and watermelon daikon radish, substitute shredded red beets and sliced radishes. This vegetable slaw can also be rolled up in a gluten-free tortilla or softened rice paper for a quick wrap, or top it with cooked grains or gluten-free pasta for a hearty one-plate meal.

DEFINITION

Watermelon daikon radishes are round like a beet and have a similar appearance to their namesake, with a light green outer skin and bright pink inside. They differ from other daikon radishes, which look like a long, overly fat, large white carrot. Find them alongside other root vegetables in the produce section or at farmers' markets during the summer and fall months.

Deli-Style Coleslaw

Every deli counter seems to offer its own signature blend of coleslaw, and here's ours, made with crunchy green and red cabbages and bright carrots, tossed in a creamy, sweet, and tangy dressing made with our Reduced-Fat Soy Milk Mayo.

Yield:	Prep time:	Serving size:
6 cups	8 to 10 minutes	1 cup

4 cups cabbage, shredded

2 cups red cabbage, shredded

2 cups carrots, shredded

¼ cup green onion, thinly sliced

¼ cup chopped fresh parsley

1 cup Reduced-Fat Soy Milk Mayo
(recipe in Chapter 9)

¼ cup apple cider vinegar

2 TB. spicy brown mustard or Dijon
mustard

1½ TB. gluten-free brown rice
syrup or maple syrup

1½ tsp. celery seed

1 tsp. sea salt

½ tsp. freshly ground black pepper

1. In a large bowl, combine cabbage, red cabbage, carrots, green onion, and parsley, and toss together.

2. In a small bowl, combine Reduced-Fat Soy Milk Mayo, apple cider vinegar, spicy brown mustard, brown rice syrup, celery seed, sea salt, and pepper. Pour dressing over cabbage mixture, and stir gently until evenly coated.

3. Serve immediately or chill for 30 minutes or more to allow flavors to blend. Serve as a side salad with sandwiches or wraps.

Variation: For a **Fat-Free Sweet and Spicy Coleslaw,** omit the Reduced-Fat Soy Milk Mayo and brown rice syrup, and instead make a dressing by whisking together an additional 3 tablespoons spicy brown mustard, ⅓ cup maple syrup, 1 teaspoon onion powder, and ½ teaspoon garlic powder, along with the apple cider vinegar, celery seed, sea salt, and pepper. Pour dressing over the cabbage mixture, and toss well to combine. For extra texture, add 1½ tablespoons chia seeds or poppy seeds.

CORNUCOPIA

Curly parsley, with its fluffy, ruffled edges, is mildly sweet. Italian or flat-leaf parsley has a stronger flavor and is used more often in cooked dishes.

Sensational Sandwiches

In This Chapter

- Layered cold sandwiches
- Veganized deli-style offerings
- Hot and healthy sandwiches

Sandwiches and wraps make for great handheld meals for lunch, dinner, or whenever you're in need of a snack or a meal on the go. Whether you're hankering for a cold one or something steaming hot and juicy, you're bound to find something to your liking in the pages ahead.

Many of these recipes feature our own homemade gluten-free bread and hamburger buns, vegan cheese slices, condiments, and meatless meats from other chapters in the book. But if you don't have time to prepare these extra sandwich-building components, you can always substitute similar store-bought ingredients.

The offerings in this chapter are bound to fulfill your gluten-free vegan sandwich needs. We've got new twists on many American deli-style classics, like a meatless stacked club sandwich, tofu-based egg salad, and even a tempeh reuben. So get ready to impress your friends, family, and co-workers (who often gawk at what you're having for lunch) with some sensational-looking and -tasting sandwiches!

West Coast Club Sandwiches

We're both West Coast girls and have access to a wide assortment of fresh produce year-round. This plethora of produce inspired this vegan club sandwich, featuring stacked layers of colorful, fresh veggies and our Garnet Yam Hummus.

Yield:	Prep time:	Serving size:
4 sandwiches	15 to 20 minutes	1 sandwich

8 slices Multi-Grain Sandwich Bread (recipe in Chapter 5) or other gluten-free bread

1 cup Garnet Yam Hummus (recipe in Chapter 8)

4 large leaves red-tipped loose-leaf lettuce or other lettuce

¾ cup sweet potatoes, peeled and shredded

¾ cup zucchini, shredded

2 large Roma tomatoes, each cut into 8 slices

½ cucumber, cut into 16 thin slices

½ cup carrots, shredded

1 cup Fresh and Flavorful Sprouts using red clover (recipe in Chapter 10) or other fresh sprouts

1. To assemble sandwiches, toast slices of Multi-Grain Sandwich Bread (if desired) and place on a large cutting board or work surface. Spread 2 tablespoons Garnet Yam Hummus on each piece of bread.

2. Top 4 bread slices each with 1 lettuce leaf. Evenly layer, in this order, 3 tablespoons sweet potatoes, 3 tablespoons zucchini, 4 Roma tomato slices, 4 cucumber slices, 2 tablespoons carrots, and ¼ cup Fresh and Flavorful Sprouts using red clover.

3. Place remaining 4 slices of Multi-Grain Sandwich Bread on top of vegetables, hummus side in, and gently press down on each sandwich. Carefully slice sandwiches diagonally in half. Serve immediately, or place them in an airtight container or wrap them tightly in plastic wrap and store in the refrigerator for up to 2 days.

Variation: Feel free to replace the Garnet Yam Hummus with Dijon or spicy brown mustard, Reduced-Fat Soy Milk Mayo (recipe in Chapter 9), or another spread as desired.

MEATLESS AND WHEATLESS

To amp up your plate presentation, use frilly toothpicks to secure your layered sandwiches. This also makes it easier for you to cut them diagonally in half.

BBQ Seitan 'n' Slaw Sandwiches

Our love of spicy food drove us to create this meatless version of pulled-pork sandwiches, which we've assembled with sauce-covered strips of gluten-free seitan, topped with a little creamy coleslaw and sprouts to offset the heat of the fiery BBQ sauce.

Yield:	Prep time:	Cook time:	Serving size:
4 sandwiches	10 to 12 minutes	10 to 15 minutes	1 sandwich

2 cups Beef-Style Gluten-Free Seitan (variation in Chapter 12), cut into ¼-in.-thick strips

1 cup Bourbon Blues BBQ Sauce (recipe in Chapter 9)

4 Gluten-Free Hamburger Buns (recipe in Chapter 5), split

1 cup Deli-Style Coleslaw (recipe in Chapter 10)

1 cup Fresh and Flavorful Sprouts using alfalfa (recipe in Chapter 10), or other fresh sprouts

1. Preheat the oven to 350°F. Lightly oil a 9-inch baking pan.

2. In a medium bowl, combine Beef-Style Gluten-Free Seitan strips and Bourbon Blues BBQ Sauce. Transfer to the prepared baking pan. Bake for 10 to 15 minutes or until heated through. Remove from the oven.

3. To assemble sandwiches, place 4 bottom halves of Gluten-Free Hamburger Buns on a large cutting board or work surface. Place ½ cup seitan strips mixture on bottom buns, ¼ cup Deli-Style Coleslaw, ¼ cup Fresh and Flavorful Sprouts using alfalfa, and replace top halves of buns. Serve immediately.

Variation: You can replace the seitan strips mixture with Soy BBQ Slices or Soy BBQ "Short Ribs" (recipe in Chapter 12), using for each sandwich either 1 large piece of tofu (or 2 pieces of tempeh) or 4 short ribs strips.

AGAINST THE GRAIN

Barbecue sauce (as well as other tomato-based sauces) can really stain your clothes, so we suggest tying a napkin around your neck, in addition to having plenty of napkins nearby when you hunker down to eat one of these saucy sandwiches. They're messy to eat, but oh so good!

Florentine Veggie Burgers

Most store-bought veggie burgers are made with mainly soy products, but not these. These tasty oven-baked burgers are made with a savory blend of cashews, kale, mushrooms, and other vegetables.

Yield:	Prep time:	Cook time:	Serving size:
6 burgers	10 to 15 minutes	35 to 40 minutes	1 burger

2 or 3 slices Multi-Grain Sandwich Bread (recipe in Chapter 5)

1½ cups lacinato (Italian) kale or other greens, stems removed, roughly chopped, and tightly packed

⅓ cup green onion, thinly sliced

1 cup crimini mushrooms or other mushrooms, roughly chopped

¾ cup carrots, diced

¾ cup celery, diced

¾ cup yellow or red onion, diced

½ cup raw cashews

¼ cup low-sodium vegetable broth

¼ cup chopped fresh parsley

2 TB. nutritional yeast flakes

¾ tsp. sea salt

1½ tsp. Italian seasoning blend, or ½ tsp. each dried basil, oregano, and thyme

½ tsp. smoked paprika or sweet paprika

½ tsp. freshly ground black pepper or garlic pepper

¼ tsp. chili powder

¼ tsp. poultry seasoning blend

⅓ cup chickpea/garbanzo bean flour

6 Gluten-Free Hamburger Buns (recipe in Chapter 5), split

Lettuce leaves, tomato slices, slices Mellow Jack or Better Cheddar Cheese (recipes in Chapter 6), pickle slices, or toppings of choice

Reduced-Fat Soy Milk Mayo (recipe in Chapter 9), mustard, ketchup, or condiments of choice

1. In a food processor fitted with an S blade, place Multi-Grain Sandwich Bread slices, and process for 1 minute or until you get fine crumbs. Measure out 1½ cups breadcrumbs (save any extra for use in another recipe), place on a large plate, and set aside to dry out while preparing remaining burger ingredients.

2. Place a medium, nonstick skillet over medium heat. Add lacinato kale and green onion, and cook, stirring often, for 2 or 3 minutes or until wilted. Transfer to a small plate, and set aside.

3. Return the skillet to the heat. Add crimini mushrooms, and cook, stirring often, for 2 or 3 minutes to remove excess moisture. Remove from heat.

4. Place carrots, celery, yellow onion, and cashews in the food processor, and process for 1 or 2 minutes or until finely ground. Scrape down the sides of the container with a spatula and process for 30 more seconds.

5. Transfer carrot mixture to a large bowl. Add reserved kale mixture, mushrooms, and breadcrumbs, along with vegetable broth, parsley, nutritional yeast flakes, sea salt, Italian seasoning blend, smoked paprika, pepper, chili powder, and poultry seasoning blend, and stir well to combine. Stir in chickpea/garbanzo bean flour.

6. Preheat the oven to 425°F. Line a cookie sheet with parchment paper or a Silpat liner.

7. Using a $\frac{1}{2}$ cup measuring cup to portion each burger patty, lightly fill and gently pack burger mixture into the measuring cup with the back of a spoon. Flip over patty onto the prepared cookie sheet, and give the measuring cup a tap to release patty. Repeat with remaining burger mixture to make 6 patties. Using a burger press or your hands, slightly flatten patties.

8. Bake for 15 minutes. Remove from the oven. Flip over patties with a spatula. Return to the oven, and bake for 10 to 15 more minutes or until golden brown. Serve burgers on Gluten-Free Hamburger Buns with your choice of toppings and condiments.

Variation: You can chill the patties for 30 minutes and then cook them in a large, nonstick skillet with a little olive oil for 2 or 3 minutes per side or until lightly browned.

MEATLESS AND WHEATLESS

By using a $\frac{1}{2}$ cup measuring cup, you can easily portion out quarter-pounder-size veggie burgers, which then just need to be flattened a bit with either your hands or a burger press. You can find burger presses in kitchen supply stores. They consist of a large ring and hand-grip plunger, which helps you form uniformly sized and well-compacted patties.

Hot S.M.O. Sandwiches

These hot sandwiches feature three main ingredients—spinach, mushrooms, and onions (S.M.O.)—which are quickly sautéed together to create a sensational savory sandwich.

Yield:	Prep time:	Cook time:	Serving size:
2 sandwiches	5 to 7 minutes	5 to 7 minutes	1 sandwich

2/3 cup crimini mushrooms or other mushrooms, cut in 1/2 and thinly sliced

2/3 cup red onion, cut into 1/2 moons

1 1/2 tsp. olive oil

1 TB. garlic, minced

1/2 tsp. dried basil

1/4 tsp. crushed red pepper flakes

1/8 tsp. freshly ground black pepper

1 bunch spinach, washed well and stems removed, or 6 cups baby spinach, tightly packed

1/2 tsp. wheat-free tamari

1/2 tsp. balsamic vinegar (optional)

4 slices Multi-Grain Sandwich Bread (recipe in Chapter 5) or other gluten-free bread

1. Place a large, nonstick skillet over medium heat. Add crimini mushrooms, red onion, and olive oil, and sauté, stirring often, for 3 or 4 minutes or until soft and slightly browned.

2. Add garlic, basil, crushed red pepper flakes, and pepper, and sauté, stirring often, for 1 more minute.

3. Add spinach, tamari, and balsamic vinegar (if using), and sauté, stirring often, for 1 or 2 more minutes or until spinach begins to wilt. Remove from heat.

4. To assemble sandwiches, toast slices of Multi-Grain Sandwich Bread (if desired), and place on a large cutting board or work surface. Evenly divide spinach mixture between top 2 bread slices, and place remaining slices of bread on top. Slice each sandwich in half, and serve.

Variation: For extra flavor, spread Basil, Spinach, and Pumpkin Seed Pesto (recipe in Chapter 9), Garnet Yam Hummus (recipe in Chapter 8), or a little Reduced-Fat Soy Milk Mayo (recipe in Chapter 9) on bread slices as desired prior to assembling sandwiches. Feel free to replace the spinach with other varieties of greens, such as arugula, kale, or Swiss chard, as well as add slices of Mellow Jack Cheese (recipe in Chapter 6) or tomatoes.

Plant-Based Dietitian Recommends: Substitute 2 tablespoons vegetable broth or water for the oil.

> **AGAINST THE GRAIN**
>
> There's nothing worse than biting into a dish or salad that features fresh greens and feeling the slight crunch of dirt or grit between your teeth. To avoid grit in your greens, wash them in cold water several times, a procedure referred to as "triple washing." You can rinse your greens in a colander under running water several times, but we prefer to submerge them in a bowl full of water, lift out the greens, place them into a colander, and repeat the process as needed. The dirt will sink to the bottom of the bowl.

Tempeh Reubens

These tasty, meat-free reubens are made with our Smoky Tempeh Un-Bacon and Better Cheddar cheese, some sautéed sauerkraut, and a quick and easy Thousand Island Dressing. For a deli-style meal, serve them alongside potato salad or coleslaw and a pickle spear.

Yield:	Prep time:	Cook time:	Serving size:
4 sandwiches	10 to 15 minutes	7 to 10 minutes	1 sandwich

1 cup sauerkraut, drained

1 TB. olive oil

1/4 tsp. caraway seeds

1/4 tsp. freshly ground black pepper or garlic pepper

8 slices Smoky Tempeh Un-Bacon (recipe in Chapter 12)

4 slices Better Cheddar or Mellow Jack Cheese (recipes in Chapter 6)

1/2 cup Reduced-Fat Soy Milk Mayo (recipe in Chapter 9)

1/4 cup ketchup

1 1/2 TB. prepared pickle relish

8 slices Multi-Grain Sandwich Bread (recipe in Chapter 5) or other gluten-free bread

1. Place a large, nonstick skillet over medium heat. Add sauerkraut, 1 1/2 teaspoons olive oil, caraway seeds, and pepper, and sauté, stirring often, for 3 to 5 minutes or until dry and slightly browned. Transfer sauerkraut to a small plate, and set aside.

2. Return the skillet to medium heat. Add Smoky Tempeh Un-Bacon and remaining $1\frac{1}{2}$ teaspoons olive oil, and cook for 2 minutes. Flip over Smoky Tempeh Un-Bacon with a spatula, and cook for 2 or 3 more minutes or until heated through.

3. Group Smoky Tempeh Un-Bacon into pairs, place 1 slice Better Cheddar on top of each pair, cover the skillet, cook for 1 minute, and remove from heat.

4. In a small bowl, combine Reduced-Fat Soy Milk Mayo, ketchup, and pickle relish.

5. To assemble reubens, toast slices of Multi-Grain Sandwich Bread and place them on a large cutting board or work surface. Evenly divide dressing and spread on each slice of bread. Top 4 bread slices with cheese-covered tempeh pairs, and equally divide sauerkraut mixture over tempeh. Top with remaining slices of bread. Slice each sandwich in half, and serve.

Variation: For **Avocado Reubens,** replace the Smoky Tempeh Un-Bacon on each sandwich with $\frac{1}{4}$ of sliced Hass avocado and 2 slices tomato.

Plant-Based Dietitian Recommends: Substitute 4 tablespoons vegetable broth or water for the oil, separated into 2 tablespoons for steps 1 and 2.

MEATLESS AND WHEATLESS

We've opted to toast our slices of bread and then assemble our reuben sandwiches, but you can go another route if you like. Assemble the sandwiches using untoasted bread, lightly oil the previously used large skillet, and cook the sandwiches for 2 or 3 minutes per side or until lightly browned. Or if you have one, cook them in a panini sandwich maker or other hinged countertop grilling machine.

Sloppy Janes

We developed this hearty, mildly seasoned, tempeh-based Sloppy Janes recipe for all the gluten-free vegan kids out there. (Adults will enjoy them, too!)

Yield:	Prep time:	Cook time:	Serving size:
6 sandwiches	10 minutes	10 minutes	1 sandwich

1 (8-oz.) pkg. tempeh, cut into
   ½-in. cubes

1 TB. olive oil

5 TB. low-sodium vegetable broth

½ cup red onion, diced

½ cup green bell pepper, diced

½ cup red bell pepper, diced

2 TB. jalapeño pepper, ribs and
   seeds removed, and finely diced

1½ TB. garlic, minced

1 cup fire-roasted crushed
   tomatoes

1 TB. nutritional yeast flakes

1 tsp. wheat-free tamari

1 tsp. dried oregano

1 tsp. chili powder

½ tsp. *smoked paprika* or sweet
   paprika

¼ tsp. freshly ground black pepper

6 Gluten-Free Hamburger Buns
   (recipe in Chapter 4), split

1. Place a large, nonstick skillet over medium heat. Add tempeh cubes and olive oil, and sauté, stirring often, for 2 minutes. Add 3 tablespoons vegetable broth, and cook, stirring often, for 3 more minutes.

2. Add red onion, green bell pepper, red bell pepper, jalapeño pepper, garlic, and remaining 2 tablespoons vegetable broth, and cook, stirring often, for 3 more minutes.

3. Add crushed tomatoes, nutritional yeast flakes, tamari, oregano, chili powder, smoked paprika, and pepper, and cook, stirring often, for 2 more minutes. Remove from heat.

4. Evenly divide mixture among Gluten-Free Hamburger Buns, and serve hot.

Variation: For milder-flavored Sloppy Janes, replace the fire-roasted crushed tomatoes with ¾ cup ketchup and 1 tablespoon spicy brown mustard or 1 (6-ounce) can tomato paste and ⅓ cup water. To adapt this recipe into a baked casserole,

Tempeh–Corn Chip Pie, place the Sloppy Janes mixture in a lightly oiled 9-inch baking pan. Top with 1½ cups corn chips or tortilla chips (crumbled a bit with your fingers) and ¾ cup Cheesy Sauce (recipe in Chapter 6). Bake at 400°F for 10 to 15 minutes or until Cheesy Sauce is bubbly, and serve hot.

Plant-Based Dietitian Recommends: Substitute an additional 2 tablespoons vegetable broth or water for the oil, for a total of 7 tablespoons vegetable broth or water.

> **DEFINITION**
>
> **Smoked paprika** is a variety of Spanish paprika made from mature pimento peppers that are dried, naturally smoked over oak wood fires, and stone-ground to a fine, powdery consistency. It has a deep red color with a slightly smoky and bittersweet flavor and is available in most grocery and natural foods stores, as well as through online sources.

Deviled Eggless Egg Salad Wraps

This zesty tofu- and veggie-based spread is generously seasoned and tinted by chili and curry powders.

Yield:	Prep time:	Serving size:
6 wraps	10 minutes, plus 30 minutes chill time	1 wrap

8 oz. firm or extra-firm tofu

1½ TB. nutritional yeast flakes

1½ TB. lemon juice

1½ TB. Dijon mustard

1 TB. wheat-free tamari

2 tsp. onion powder

2 tsp. garlic powder or garlic granules

1½ tsp. curry powder

1 tsp. chili powder or smoked paprika

1 tsp. celery seed

1 tsp. sea salt

¼ tsp. freshly ground black pepper

¼ cup Reduced-Fat Soy Milk Mayo (recipe in Chapter 9)

3 TB. celery, finely diced

3 TB. red bell pepper, finely diced

3 TB. carrots, shredded

3 TB. chopped fresh parsley

2 TB. green onion, thinly sliced

1 TB. prepared pickle relish

6 (8-in.) brown rice, hemp, or other gluten-free tortillas

6 large leaves red-tipped loose-leaf lettuce or other lettuce

2 large Roma tomatoes, each cut into 6 slices

1½ cups Fresh and Flavorful Sprouts using alfalfa (recipe in Chapter 10), or other fresh sprouts

1. Using your fingers, crumble tofu into a medium bowl. Add nutritional yeast flakes, lemon juice, Dijon mustard, tamari, onion powder, garlic powder, curry powder, chili powder, celery seed, sea salt, and pepper. Using a potato masher, mash together tofu and seasonings until well combined. Cover and chill for 15 minutes.

2. Add Reduced-Fat Soy Milk Mayo, celery, red bell pepper, carrots, parsley, green onion, and pickle relish, and stir well to combine. Cover and chill for 15 minutes to allow flavors to blend.

3. For easier rolling, warm each tortilla in a large skillet over medium heat for 1 or 2 minutes per side, or warm in a microwave oven for 20 to 30 seconds.

4. To assemble each wrap, place 1 warmed tortilla on a large cutting board or work surface. Place 1 lettuce leaf vertically in the center of tortilla so it hangs slightly over top edge. In the center of lettuce leaf, place $\frac{1}{6}$ of eggless egg mixture (approximately a generous $\frac{1}{2}$ cup), and top with 2 Roma tomato slices and $\frac{1}{4}$ cup Fresh and Flavorful Sprouts using alfalfa.

5. Fold bottom half of tortilla up to the center, and fold in each side, one overlapping the other, to partially enclose filling ingredients. Secure wrap with a toothpick, threading it through both sides. Serve immediately, or wrap tightly in plastic wrap and place in an airtight container. Stored in the refrigerator, wraps will keep for up to 2 or 3 days.

Variation: If wraps aren't your thing, you can also assemble the Deviled Eggless Egg Salad and veggie components on slices of Multi-Grain Sandwich Bread (recipe in Chapter 5) or serve as an open-faced sandwich on toasted gluten-free English muffins.

CORNUCOPIA

The average large egg contains 212 milligrams cholesterol. Fortunately for us vegans, plant-based foods are all cholesterol free!

Meatless Meats

In This Chapter

- Meat-free bacons and sausages
- Gluten-free seitan
- Soy-based cutlets and cubes

Fortunately for vegans, most grocery and natural foods stores these days stock several varieties of meatless meats, but many of them contain gluten-based flours or by-products. We're here to show you how to make your own delicious, nutritious meatless meat alternatives.

For all you vegans who heartily enjoyed seitan-based dishes prior to going gluten free—surprise! We've developed several gluten-free seitan selections made with brown rice, chickpea, and soy flours, rather than the typical whole-wheat flour and vital wheat gluten. They're just as firm, chewy, and meatlike in texture as wheat-based seitan.

And if you're a tofu and tempeh lover, you've come to the right place. In this chapter, we share several suggestions for covering these soy-based products with savory sauces, marinades, and breading mixtures to bake some magnificent meat-free options you can enjoy as is or add to recipes.

Smoky Tempeh Un-Bacon

A full-flavored marinade of sweet apple juice, apple cider vinegar, and maple syrup, plus a blend of smoked paprika, chipotle chili powder, and a bit of *smoked sea salt* coats these thin slices of oven-baked tempeh.

Yield:	Prep time:	Cook time:	Serving size:
8 slices	5 minutes, plus 1 hour or more marinate time	25 to 30 minutes	2 slices

1 (8-oz.) pkg. tempeh

2 TB. wheat-free tamari

1 TB. apple juice or water

1 TB. apple cider vinegar

1 TB. maple syrup

1 tsp. toasted sesame oil or olive oil

½ tsp. smoked paprika

½ tsp. chipotle chili powder or chili powder

½ tsp. garlic powder or garlic granules

¼ tsp. freshly ground black pepper or garlic pepper

¼ tsp. smoked sea salt or liquid smoke flavoring

1. Cut tempeh block into quarters lengthwise, and slice each piece horizontally to yield 8 pieces. Place tempeh slices on a large plate.

2. In a small bowl, combine tamari, apple juice, apple cider vinegar, maple syrup, toasted sesame oil, smoked paprika, chipotle chili powder, garlic powder, pepper, and smoked sea salt.

3. Drizzle ½ of marinade mixture over tempeh slices, flip over slices, and drizzle remaining marinade mixture over slices. Chill tempeh and leave to marinate for 1 hour or more as desired.

4. Preheat the oven to 400°F. Line a cookie sheet with parchment paper or a Silpat liner.

5. Place tempeh slices on the prepared cookie sheet, and spoon any remaining marinade over tempeh slices. Bake for 15 minutes. Remove from the oven, flip over tempeh slices with a spatula, and bake for 10 to 15 more minutes or until golden brown and crisp around the edges. Serve hot. Store tempeh slices in an airtight container in the refrigerator for up to 1 week.

Variation: This recipe can also be prepared with 8 ounces firm or extra-firm tofu instead.

Plant-Based Dietitian Recommends: Omit the oil and monitor the cook time, which may be a few minutes shorter, to prevent burning.

DEFINITION

Smoked sea salt is made from sea salt that's been slow-smoked for several hours over various types of wood, such as hickory, mesquite, or alder. It has a full-bodied, very intense, smoky flavor and aroma and is often used as a replacement for liquid smoke flavoring to add a bit of smokiness to barbecue sauces, marinades, dry rubs, and grilled or oven-roasted items.

Savory Sausages

We've combined white beans and several gluten-free flours and starches with some of our favorite go-to condiments, herbs, and spices to create these tasty meatless sausages.

Yield:	Prep time:	Cook time:	Serving size:
8 (5-inch) sausages	15 to 20 minutes, plus 25 minutes rest time	30 minutes steam time	1 sausage

¾ cup brown rice flour

¾ cup chickpea/garbanzo bean flour

6 TB. soy flour

6 TB. tapioca starch

2 TB. nutritional yeast flakes

1 tsp. dried basil

1 tsp. dried oregano

1 tsp. rubbed sage

1 tsp. onion powder

1 tsp. garlic powder or garlic granules

1 tsp. chili powder

1 tsp. smoked paprika

½ tsp. sea salt

½ tsp. freshly ground black pepper or garlic pepper

⅓ cup canned Great Northern beans or other white bean, drained and rinsed

¾ cup low-sodium vegetable broth

1½ TB. wheat-free tamari

1½ TB. ketchup

1½ TB. maple syrup

1. Set up a large pot with a collapsible steamer basket or a steamer rack insert. Add enough water so it just touches the bottom of collapsible steamer or is 1 or 2 inches deep if using rack insert. Cover the pot, and bring to a boil over medium heat.

2. In a large bowl, combine brown rice flour, chickpea/garbanzo bean flour, soy flour, tapioca starch, nutritional yeast flakes, basil, oregano, sage, onion powder, garlic powder, chili powder, smoked paprika, sea salt, and pepper.

3. In a medium bowl, place Great Northern beans. Using a potato masher, mash beans until smooth. Stir in vegetable broth, tamari, ketchup, and maple syrup. Add wet ingredients to dry ingredients, and stir well to combine.

4. Cut 8 (6×8-inch) pieces of parchment paper and aluminum foil. In an assembly line fashion, on a work surface, place parchment papers on top of pieces of aluminum foil.

5. Using a ¼ cup measuring cup, portion sausage mixture, and place each portion lengthwise in the center of the parchment paper. Using your hands, shape each portion into a 5-inch log. Fold over edges of the parchment paper to enclose sausage log. Roll up aluminum foil to enclose sausage log, and twist ends to secure (like a Tootsie Roll).

6. Place sausages in the steamer, and steam for 30 minutes. Turn off the steamer, and let sausages sit in the steamer for 5 more minutes. Remove sausages from the steamer, place on a large plate, and set aside to cool for 20 minutes.

7. Serve immediately or refrigerate until ready to eat. Serve sausages with your favorite breakfast items (see recipes in Chapter 4), as a side dish with savory entrées or other dishes, or sliced or chopped in recipes as desired. Store sausages in an airtight container or zipper-lock bag in the refrigerator for up to 5 days, or freeze for up to 3 months.

Variation: To make larger sausages for serving in buns as sandwiches, portion sausage mixture with ½ cup measuring cup, and use 4 (6×12-inch) pieces of parchment paper and aluminum foil. Also, if you prefer a crispy outer crust on your sausages, after they've been steamed, cook them in a lightly oiled, large, nonstick skillet for several minutes or until browned on all sides.

AGAINST THE GRAIN

In the past few years, aluminum-based cookware and foil have been linked to Alzheimer's disease. In an effort to reduce such unnecessary health risks, many chefs and other food professionals have chosen to limit direct contact of the foods we prepare with aluminum foil. That's the reason for the layer of parchment paper between food items and aluminum foil.

Chicken-Style Gluten-Free Seitan

Seitan (a.k.a. wheat meat) is no longer off limits for gluten-free vegans! With the help of some veggies, nutritional yeast, and seasonings, our seitan even has a chicken-y flavor.

Yield:	Prep time:	Cook time:	Serving size:
1 (9-inch) log or 1½ pounds	15 to 20 minutes, plus 25 minutes rest time	8 to 10 minutes, plus 1 hour steam time	¾ cup

1¼ cups low-sodium vegetable broth

¼ cup carrots, finely diced

¼ cup celery, finely diced

¼ cup yellow onion, finely diced

2 TB. garlic, minced

6 TB. firm or extra-firm tofu

3 TB. wheat-free tamari

½ cup brown rice flour

½ cup chickpea/garbanzo bean flour

½ cup soy flour

¼ cup tapioca starch

½ cup nutritional yeast flakes

4 tsp. onion powder

4 tsp. garlic powder or garlic granules

4 tsp. *poultry seasoning blend*

2 tsp. dried thyme

1 tsp. sea salt

½ tsp. freshly ground black pepper

1. Place a medium, nonstick skillet over medium heat. Add ½ cup vegetable broth, carrots, celery, yellow onion, and garlic, and cook, stirring often, for 8 to 10 minutes or until vegetables are tender. Remove from heat.

2. Transfer vegetable mixture to a blender or food processor fitted with an S blade. Add remaining ¾ cup vegetable broth, tofu, and tamari, and process for 1 or 2 minutes or until smooth.

3. In a large bowl, combine brown rice flour, chickpea/garbanzo bean flour, soy flour, tapioca starch, nutritional yeast flakes, onion powder, garlic powder, poultry seasoning blend, thyme, sea salt, and pepper. Add wet ingredients to dry ingredients, and stir well to combine.

4. Set up a large pot with a collapsible steamer basket or a steamer rack insert. Add enough water so it just touches the bottom of collapsible steamer or is 2 inches deep if using a rack insert. Cover the pot and bring to a boil over medium heat.

5. Cut a 12×12-inch piece of parchment paper and aluminum foil. Place the parchment paper on top of the piece of aluminum foil. Place seitan mixture lengthwise in the center of the parchment paper. Using your hands, shape mixture into a 9-inch log. Fold over the edges of the parchment paper to enclose seitan log. Roll up aluminum foil to enclose seitan log, and twist ends to secure (like a Tootsie Roll).

6. Place seitan log in the steamer, and steam for 1 hour. Turn off the steamer, and let seitan log sit in the steamer for 5 more minutes. Remove seitan from the steamer, place on a large plate, and set aside to cool for 20 minutes.

7. Serve immediately or refrigerate until ready to eat. Serve slices of seitan as a side dish with savory entrées or other dishes, use slices on sandwiches or in wraps, or add slices or chopped pieces to recipes as desired. Store seitan in an airtight container or zipper-lock bag in the refrigerator for up to 5 days, or freeze for up to 3 months.

Variation: If you prefer, you can shape the seitan mixture into 2 smaller logs and use 2 (8×12-inch) pieces of parchment paper and aluminum foil instead. To make **Beef-Style Gluten-Free Seitan,** replace the carrots and celery with 1 cup chopped crimini or other mushrooms and cook for 10 minutes, and add 3 tablespoons ketchup to the blended wet ingredients. In the dry ingredients, only add ¼ cup nutritional yeast flakes and 2 teaspoons each onion and garlic powders, and replace the poultry seasoning blend with 2 teaspoons each dried basil and oregano.

DEFINITION

Poultry seasoning blend is made of a blend of dried herbs and spices and often includes sage, thyme, rosemary, marjoram, black pepper, and celery seed. It gets its name because many of these seasonings are used to flavor poultry. You can also use this savory seasoning blend to flavor stuffing, rice and grains, as well as vegetable-based dishes.

Miso-Glazed Tofu

This tofu is marinated in a slightly sweet, sour, and salty mix of miso, brown rice vinegar, maple syrup, and a bit of hot pepper sauce for some kick, which when baked, forms a savory glaze.

Yield:	Prep time:	Cook time:	Serving size:
16 pieces	8 to 10 minutes, plus 1 hour or more marinate time	25 to 30 minutes	2 pieces

1 lb. firm or extra-firm tofu	1 TB. garlic, minced
¼ cup maple syrup	1 TB. fresh ginger, minced
¼ cup brown rice vinegar	2 tsp. toasted sesame oil
3 TB. mellow miso or other miso	1 tsp. hot pepper sauce
2 TB. wheat-free tamari	

1. Squeeze block of tofu over the sink to remove excess water. Cut tofu in half lengthwise, turn each half cut side down, cut each half into 4 slices, and cut each slice diagonally into a triangle for a total of 16 pieces. Place tofu triangles in a 8×10-inch baking pan.

2. In a small bowl, whisk together maple syrup, brown rice vinegar, mellow miso, tamari, garlic, ginger, toasted sesame oil, and hot pepper sauce. Pour mixture over tofu in the baking pan.

3. Refrigerate for 1 hour or more to marinate. After 30 minutes of marinating, flip over tofu triangles, and place back in the refrigerator.

4. Preheat the oven to 400°F.

5. Bake for 15 minutes. Remove from the oven. Flip over tofu triangles with a spatula. Return to the oven, and bake for 10 to 15 more minutes or until golden brown. Serve hot or cold as a main or side dish with cooked vegetables, grains, gluten-free noodles, stir-fries, or your other favorite Asian dishes.

Variation: For a firmer texture, use pressed or frozen and thawed tofu, or replace the firm tofu with super firm tofu.

Plant-Based Dietitian Recommends: Omit the oil and monitor the cook time, which may be a few minutes shorter, to prevent burning.

> **MEATLESS AND WHEATLESS**
>
> For a firmer and chewier texture, freeze your block of tofu, either in the package it came in or in an airtight container or zipper-lock bag, until solid. Then, allow it to thaw overnight in the refrigerator. If you're in a hurry, submerge it in warm water for 30 minutes or as needed. The freezing and thawing process brings out the tofu's spongelike qualities. Give the block a good squeeze to release the excess moisture before using it in your recipe.

Soy BBQ "Short Ribs"

Ready for some lip-smackin' good vegan BBQ? In less than an hour, you can make and bake these saucy, meatless "short ribs," made with strips of tofu covered in our smoky and spicy Bourbon Blues BBQ Sauce.

Yield:	Prep time:	Cook time:	Serving size:
16 strips	5 to 7 minutes	35 to 40 minutes	4 strips

1 lb. extra-firm or super firm tofu
  or 2 (8-oz.) pkg. tempeh
1 TB. olive oil

1 TB. wheat-free tamari
1 cup Bourbon Blues BBQ Sauce
  (recipe in Chapter 9)

1. Preheat the oven to 350°F. Lightly oil a 8×10-inch baking pan.

2. Cut block of tofu into half lengthwise, turn each half cut side down, cut each half into 4 slices, and then cut each slice in half lengthwise to yield a total of 16 pieces. (If using tempeh, cut each package of tempeh into 8 pieces.)

3. Place tofu pieces in a single layer in the prepared baking pan.

4. In a small bowl, combine olive oil and tamari. Pour mixture over tofu pieces. Flip over each piece to evenly coat on all sides.

5. Bake for 20 minutes. Remove from the oven. Flip over pieces with a spatula. Spread Bourbon Blues BBQ Sauce evenly over pieces, and bake for 15 to 20 more minutes or until sauce is bubbly. Remove from the oven.

6. Serve 4 strips per person, hot or cold as desired, as a side or main dish; on buns as a sandwich filling; or chop and use to add flavor to soups, stews, or grains.

Variation: Feel free to replace the Bourbon Blues BBQ Sauce with store-bought bottled barbecue sauce (just be alert for gluten when reading the ingredient list). For large **Soy BBQ Slices,** cut the block of tofu in half lengthwise, turn each half cut side down, and cut each half into 4 slices to yield a total of 8 pieces. Top with olive oil–tamari mixture, bake, and cover with BBQ sauce as described. For **Smothered Soy Strips,** replace Bourbon Blues BBQ Sauce with Roasted Onion and Garlic Gravy (recipe in Chapter 9).

Plant-Based Dietitian Recommends: Substitute an extra 1 tablespoon wheat-free tamari or 1 tablespoon vegetable broth for the 1 tablespoon oil.

CORNUCOPIA

The most basic blocks of tempeh are made from soybeans, but you can also purchase it with other ingredients added such as different legumes, grains, vegetables, and herbs and seasonings. So be sure to check the ingredients label because not all varieties are gluten free. Some of our favorite gluten-free flavored varieties include multi-grain, wild rice, flax, garden veggie, curried lentil, and Mexican.

Pumpkin Seed–Crusted Cutlets

Pumpkin seeds add extra crunchiness, flavor, and a nutritional boost to the seasoned breading mixture that coats this tofu. These cutlets are excellent on their own, used on sandwiches, or covered with gravy for a vegan turkey alternative.

Yield:	Prep time:	Cook time:	Serving size:
8 pieces	25 to 30 minutes, plus 1 hour or more marinate time	40 to 45 minutes	2 pieces

1 lb. firm or extra-firm tofu or 2 (8-oz.) pkg. tempeh

$\frac{1}{2}$ cup soy milk or other nondairy milk

2 tsp. wheat-free tamari

1 tsp. lemon juice

$1\frac{1}{2}$ tsp. garlic powder or garlic granules

$1\frac{1}{2}$ tsp. onion powder

1 slice Multi-Grain Sandwich Bread (recipe in Chapter 5) or other gluten-free bread

$\frac{1}{3}$ cup raw pumpkin seeds

6 TB. chickpea/garbanzo bean flour

$1\frac{1}{2}$ TB. nutritional yeast flakes

$1\frac{1}{2}$ tsp. dried basil

$\frac{1}{2}$ tsp. dried thyme

$\frac{1}{2}$ tsp. chili powder

$\frac{1}{2}$ tsp. smoked paprika

$\frac{1}{4}$ tsp. sea salt

$\frac{1}{4}$ tsp. freshly ground black pepper or garlic pepper

1. Squeeze block of tofu over the sink to remove excess water. Place tofu in a colander in the sink, cover with a plate, place a 28-ounce can on top of the plate, and leave tofu to press for 20 minutes.

2. Cut pressed tofu in half lengthwise, turn each half cut side down, and cut each half into 4 slices for a total of 8 slices. (If using tempeh, cut each package of tempeh into 4 pieces.)

3. Place tofu pieces in a single layer in a 8×10-inch baking pan. Using a fork, pierce each piece of tofu several times along its length, flip over pieces, and pierce other side.

4. In a small bowl, combine soy milk, tamari, lemon juice, $\frac{1}{2}$ teaspoon garlic powder, and $\frac{1}{2}$ teaspoon onion powder. Pour mixture over tofu pieces, and flip over each piece to evenly coat on all sides. Refrigerate for 1 hour or more to marinate.

5. Meanwhile, in a food processor fitted with an S blade, place Multi-Grain Sandwich Bread slice, and process for 1 minute or until you get fine crumbs. Measure out $\frac{1}{3}$ cup breadcrumbs (save any extra for use in another recipe), place on a large plate, and set aside to dry out while preparing remaining breading ingredients.

6. Preheat the oven to 400°F. Line a cookie sheet with parchment paper or a Silpat liner, and set aside.

7. Place pumpkin seeds in a small pie pan or baking dish, and bake for 3 to 5 minutes or until lightly toasted. Remove from the oven, and let cool for 5 minutes.

8. Place toasted pumpkin seeds in the food processor, and process for 1 or 2 minutes or until finely ground. Add reserved breadcrumbs, chickpea/garbanzo bean flour, nutritional yeast flakes, basil, thyme, remaining 1 teaspoon garlic powder, remaining 1 teaspoon onion powder, chili powder, smoked paprika, sea salt, and pepper, and process for 30 seconds to combine. Transfer breading mixture to a large plate.

9. To bread cutlets, place them into breading mixture one at a time, pressing down slightly and flipping over as needed to evenly coat pieces on all sides. Place breaded pieces on the prepared cookie sheet.

10. Bake for 20 minutes. Remove from the oven. Flip over pieces with a spatula. Bake for 15 to 20 more minutes or until golden brown. Remove from the oven. Serve 2 pieces per person, hot or cold as desired.

Variation: Alternatively, you can cook tofu cutlets in batches in a little olive oil in a large, nonstick skillet for 2 or 3 minutes per side or until golden brown and crispy.

MEATLESS AND WHEATLESS

You're often told to press tofu by placing a weight on top of it for a certain period of time. This pressing procedure only adds a little extra time to your recipe prep time, but this extra step removes excess water from the tofu, giving it a denser texture, and enables the tofu to absorb more of the marinade or sauce in a recipe, which makes for a tastier final dish as well.

Baked Chickenless Nuggets

Just like some Southern cooks do, we soak our tofu nuggets in a seasoned soy butter-milk mixture for an hour and then coat them with a cornflake-based breading mixture. The nuggets bake up just as crispy as can be—and without frying.

Yield:	Prep time:	Cook time:	Serving size:
2 cups	25 to 30 minutes, plus 1 hour or more marinate time	25 to 30 minutes	$\frac{1}{2}$ cup

1 lb. firm or extra-firm tofu

$\frac{1}{2}$ cup soy milk or other nondairy milk

$1\frac{1}{2}$ TB. wheat-free tamari

$2\frac{1}{2}$ tsp. garlic powder or garlic granules

$2\frac{1}{2}$ tsp. onion powder

$\frac{1}{2}$ tsp. lemon juice

4 cups cornflakes

$\frac{1}{4}$ cup chickpea/garbanzo bean flour

2 TB. nutritional yeast flakes

1 tsp. poultry seasoning blend

1 tsp. chili powder

1 tsp. smoked paprika

$\frac{1}{4}$ tsp. sea salt

$\frac{1}{4}$ tsp. freshly ground black pepper or garlic pepper

1. Squeeze block of tofu over the sink to remove excess water. Place tofu in a colander in the sink, cover with a plate, place a 28-ounce can on top of the plate, and leave tofu to press for 20 minutes.

2. Cut pressed tofu into 1-inch cubes. Place tofu cubes in a single layer in a 8×10-inch baking pan.

3. In a small bowl, combine soy milk, tamari, $1\frac{1}{2}$ teaspoons garlic powder, $1\frac{1}{2}$ teaspoons onion powder, and lemon juice. Pour mixture over tofu cubes. Flip over each piece to evenly coat on all sides. Refrigerate for 1 hour or more to marinate.

4. Meanwhile, in a food processor fitted with an S blade, place cornflakes, chickpea/garbanzo bean flour, nutritional yeast flakes, remaining 1 teaspoon garlic powder, remaining 1 teaspoon onion powder, poultry seasoning blend, chili powder, smoked paprika, sea salt, and pepper, and process for 1 minute or until you get coarse meal. Transfer breading mixture to a large plate.

5. Preheat the oven to 400°F. Line a cookie sheet with parchment paper or a Silpat liner, and set aside.

6. To bread tofu cubes, place them into breading mixture one at a time, pressing down slightly and flipping over as needed to evenly coat pieces on all sides. With one hand, dip each tofu cube back into soy buttermilk mixture, and with your other hand, place tofu cube back in breading mixture to evenly coat on all sides one final time. Place breaded tofu cubes on the prepared cookie sheet.

7. Bake for 25 to 30 minutes or until golden brown and crispy. Remove from the oven. Serve hot with ketchup, Maple-Mustard Sauce (variation follows), or other condiments as desired.

Variation: For chewier nuggets, use frozen and thawed tofu. To make a tasty **Maple-Mustard Sauce,** stir together 3 tablespoons maple syrup and 3 tablespoons spicy brown or Dijon mustard. This is great for dipping your chickenless nuggets or raw veggies into and can also serve as salad dressing.

AGAINST THE GRAIN

Tofu and other whole soy-based products are often surrounded by confusion. Myths suggest harmful effects from their consumption. In reality, if you're getting the soy from a whole-food source (soybeans, tofu, tempeh, or even soy milk), you reap numerous health benefits. Filled with nutrients such as omega-3 fatty acids, calcium, fiber, and plant-based protein, soy products have plenty to offer. Beware of human-manipulated soy products (like soy protein isolates), widely used in processed foods and supplements. These have been found to raise harmful hormones in the blood.

Tempeh Italiano

Tangy, salty, garlicky, and spicy, and loaded with tons of flavorful herbs, this marinade mixture is packed with so much flavor, you'll find these tempeh tidbits hard to resist.

Yield:	Prep time:	Cook time:	Serving size:
2 cups	3 to 5 minutes	25 to 30 minutes	½ cup

¼ cup wheat-free tamari

2 TB. balsamic vinegar

1½ TB. garlic, minced

1½ TB. toasted sesame oil

1 TB. olive oil

1 TB. chopped fresh rosemary or 1 tsp. dried rosemary, crushed a bit with your fingers

1 TB. chopped fresh thyme or 1 tsp. dried thyme

1 tsp. dried basil

1 tsp. dried oregano

¾ tsp. ground fennel seed

½ tsp. crushed red pepper flakes

2 (8-oz.) pkg. tempeh, cut into 1-in. cubes

1. Preheat the oven to 400°F. Line a cookie sheet with parchment paper or a Silpat liner.

2. In a medium bowl, combine tamari, balsamic vinegar, garlic, toasted sesame oil, olive oil, rosemary, thyme, basil, oregano, ground fennel seed, and crushed red pepper flakes. Add tempeh cubes, and stir well to evenly coat. Transfer tempeh cubes to the prepared cookie sheet, and spread out into a single layer.

3. Bake for 15 minutes. Remove from the oven. Stir tempeh with a spatula, and spread out into a single layer again. Bake for 10 to 15 more minutes or until tempeh is golden brown around edges. Remove from the oven. Serve hot or at room temperature as desired.

Variation: For a French twist on this recipe, replace all the dried herbs with 4 teaspoons herbes de Provence. For **Tempeh Italian Cutlets,** cut each tempeh block into quarters lengthwise, place pieces in a 9×13-inch baking pan, and pour marinade over the top.

Plant-Based Dietitian Recommends: Substitute 3 tablespoons vegetable broth or water for the sesame and olive oils, but monitor the cook time to prevent burning.

CORNUCOPIA

Tempeh is created by blending cooked whole soybeans with a special culture derived from the mushroom family. When left overnight to ferment, this culture grows and binds the soybeans together, forming the mixture into a brown, flavorful cake with bits of white marbleized throughout. Those bits are why it's often considered the "blue cheese" of soy products. The fermenting process also breaks down the soybeans' protein, making it easier to digest.

Super Soups and Stews

In This Chapter

- Hot and cold tomato-based soups
- Bountiful bean and legume soups
- Thick and hearty chili, chowders, and stews

Even if you think you can't cook, you can make a pot of soup with little to no effort. Just gather some ingredients like fresh, frozen, or canned vegetables, and chop them any way you like. (The smaller the size, the faster they'll cook.) Throw them in a large pot, cover 'em up with some water or vegetable broth, and add some of your favorite herbs and spices—and maybe a bay leaf if you have one. Bring the whole shebang to a boil, cover, reduce heat to low, let it do its thing, simmering away for a half hour or more, and bim, bam, boom—you've got yourself a pot of soup. Now, wasn't that easy?

We've set you up for successful soup making in this chapter by providing instructions for making light and brothy soups, bean- and veggie-packed potfulls, thick and hearty chilis and chowders, and savory stew. Plus, making a batch of one of these will provide you with enough leftovers that you won't have to cook tomorrow, and maybe not even the day after that (depending on your and your family's appetites). It's always a great idea to keep a pot of soup stocked in your fridge to complement a meal or as a meal or snack unto itself.

Filling and nutrient-dense, soups are super staples for a healthful diet.

Edamame Gazpacho

A chunky gazpacho packed with a generous assortment of colorful and crisp garden-fresh vegetables and some shelled *edamame* for extra nutrition, this soup is perfect as a light and refreshing lunch or dinner option during the hot summer months.

Yield:	Prep time:	Serving size:
1½ quarts	15 to 20 minutes, plus 30 minutes chill time	1½ cups

3 cups tomatoes or assorted heirloom tomatoes, diced

1 (10-oz.) pkg. frozen shelled edamame, thawed

2 cups cucumber, cut into quarters lengthwise and diced

1 cup green bell pepper, diced

1 cup red, orange, or yellow bell pepper, diced

2 jalapeño peppers, ribs and seeds removed, and finely diced

½ cup green onion, thinly sliced

¼ cup chopped fresh cilantro

¼ cup chopped fresh parsley

1 TB. garlic, minced

½ tsp. Himalayan pink salt or sea salt

½ tsp. freshly ground black pepper or garlic pepper

¼ tsp. cayenne

3 cups tomato juice or vegetable juice cocktail

3 TB. red wine vinegar or balsamic vinegar

1. In a large, glass bowl, combine tomatoes, edamame, cucumber, green bell pepper, red bell pepper, jalapeño peppers, green onion, cilantro, parsley, garlic, Himalayan pink salt, pepper, and cayenne.

2. Add tomato juice and red wine vinegar, and stir gently to combine. Cover and chill for 30 minutes or more to allow flavors to blend. Taste and adjust seasonings as desired before serving.

Variation: You can replace the edamame with 1 (15-ounce) can red or black beans, drained and rinsed.

DEFINITION

Edamame are the pale green, plump, fresh soybeans that are similar in appearance to lima beans. You can typically find them packaged, both shelled or still in their protective pods, in the freezer section of your local grocery and natural foods stores. They're great added to soups, salads, stir-fries, and Asian-style noodle dishes. They're also delicious on their own as a satisfying snack.

Tex-Mex Tortilla Soup

This healthier, vegan version of the famous spicy tomato-based soup is flavored with jalapeño peppers, black beans, and corn and topped with baked tortilla strips, vegan cheese, avocado, and a little cilantro.

Yield:	Prep time:	Cook time:	Serving size:
2 quarts	10 to 15 minutes	25 to 30 minutes	1½ cups

4 (6- or 8-in.) corn tortillas

1 cup red onion, diced

3⅓ cups water or low-sodium vegetable broth

2 jalapeño peppers, ribs and seeds removed, and finely diced

2 TB. garlic, minced

2 tsp. chili powder

2 tsp. ground cumin

1 tsp. dried oregano

½ tsp. sea salt

1 (14-oz.) can fire-roasted crushed tomatoes

1 (14-oz.) can fire-roasted diced tomatoes with green chiles

1 (15-oz.) can black beans, drained and rinsed

1 cup fresh or frozen cut corn kernels

⅓ cup lime juice

Shredded Better Cheddar (recipe in Chapter 6) or other vegan cheese

1 medium Hass avocado, peeled, pitted, and diced

½ cup fresh cilantro leaves

1. Preheat the oven to 375°F. Line a large cookie sheet with parchment paper or a Silpat liner.

2. Stack tortillas on top of each other, cut in half lengthwise, and cut each half into ½-inch-wide strips. Place strips in a single layer on the prepared cookie sheet. Bake for 8 minutes or until golden and crispy. Remove from the oven, and set aside.

3. Meanwhile, in a large pot, combine red onion and ⅓ cup water, and sauté over medium heat, stirring often, for 3 minutes or until soft. Add jalapeño peppers, garlic, chili powder, cumin, oregano, and sea salt, and sauté, stirring often, for 2 more minutes.

4. Stir in remaining 3 cups water, crushed tomatoes, and diced tomatoes. Increase heat to high, and bring to a boil. Cover, reduce heat to low, and simmer for 15 minutes.

5. Remove the lid, add black beans, corn, and lime juice, and simmer for 3 more minutes. Remove from heat. Taste and adjust seasonings as desired.

6. Serve individual servings topped with a few tortilla strips, a little shredded Better Cheddar, diced Hass avocado, and cilantro leaves as desired.

Variation: Feel free to replace the canned black beans with other bean varieties. The fire-roasted tomatoes can be swapped out with regular canned tomatoes. For added bulk and flavor, you can also add 1 cup diced bell peppers or zucchini.

CORNUCOPIA

You can easily roast fresh tomatoes in your oven to give them extra flavor. Simply place halved tomatoes (or quartered larger ones) or whole cherry tomatoes in a single layer on a parchment paper– or Silpat-lined cookie sheet, and bake at 425°F for 20 to 25 minutes (depending on the size of the tomatoes) or until soft and lightly browned in several spots.

Maitake-Miso Soup

Featuring a flavorful combination of *maitake mushroom*, kombu, bok choy, and miso, this soup is as nourishing as it is filling, with its liver, colon, and cancer-fighting benefits.

Yield:	Prep time:	Cook time:	Serving size:
1½ to 2 quarts	10 minutes, plus 30 minutes or more soak time	10 minutes	1½ cups

4 (6-in.) pieces kombu	1 large stalk celery, cut in half lengthwise and thinly sliced
1 whole large dried maitake mushroom	1 TB. fresh ginger, minced
6 cups warm water	1½ TB. mellow miso or other miso
4 large leaves bok choy, collard greens, or other greens, stems trimmed or removed, and cut into fine strips	Wakame flakes or crumbled nori sheets
	Sesame seeds

1. In a 1-quart container, place kombu pieces. Into a separate 1-quart container, using your fingers, break up maitake mushroom into several pieces. Pour 3 cups warm water into each container, cover containers, and set aside for 30 minutes to allow kombu and maitake mushroom to rehydrate and soften.

2. Remove kombu and maitake mushroom from soaking liquids, transfer them to a cutting board, and set aside soaking liquids. Cut kombu into small strips, and roughly chop maitake mushroom, and place both into a large saucepan. Slowly pour both soaking liquids into the saucepan. (Discard last bit of maitake mushroom soaking liquid if it appears to have sand or debris in it.)

3. Bring to a boil over high heat, and boil for 5 minutes. Add bok choy, celery, and ginger, reduce heat to low, and simmer for 5 more minutes. Remove from heat.

4. In a small bowl, place mellow miso. Add $\frac{1}{2}$ cup hot broth from the saucepan, stir well with a spoon to dissolve miso, and stir mixture into the saucepan.

5. Top individual servings with wakame flakes and sesame seeds as desired before serving.

Variation: For a heartier soup, you can also add cubes of tofu or tempeh, buckwheat or other gluten-free noodles, cooked grains, or additional chopped vegetables of choice. Feel free to replace the dried maitake mushroom with 1 cup dried sliced shiitake mushrooms or other dried mushrooms if you like.

> **DEFINITION**
>
> **Maitake mushroom** literally means "dancing mushroom" in Japanese because, as the story goes, in ancient times, harvested maitake mushrooms could be exchanged for their weight in silver, which would in turn lead to mushroom harvesters dancing in celebration at their good fortune. These wild mushrooms, also known as "hens of the woods," have a rich, woodsy flavor and small, overlapping fan-shape caps.

Lentil and Kale Soup

Lentils and kale are a perfect pairing and seem to bring out the best in each other, flavor-wise, as this simple and satisfying soup deliciously illustrates.

Yield:	Prep time:	Cook time:	Serving size:
1½ quarts	8 to 10 minutes	40 to 45 minutes	1½ cups

6 cups water or low-sodium vegetable broth

1 cup dried brown lentils, sorted
and rinsed

1 cup carrots, diced

1 cup celery, diced

1 cup yellow onion, diced

1½ TB. garlic, minced

1 TB. herbes de Provence or Italian
seasoning blend, or 1 tsp. each
dried basil, oregano, and thyme

1 bay leaf

4 cups *lacinato* (Italian) *kale*, green
kale, or other greens, stems
removed, and roughly chopped

1 TB. nutritional yeast flakes

¾ tsp. sea salt

½ tsp. freshly ground black pepper

½ tsp. crushed red pepper flakes

1. In a large pot, combine water, lentils, carrots, celery, yellow onion, garlic, herbes de Provence, and bay leaf, and bring to a boil over high heat. Cover, reduce heat to low, and simmer for 30 minutes.

2. Add lacinato kale, nutritional yeast flakes, sea salt, pepper, and crushed red pepper flakes, and cook, stirring occasionally, for 10 to 15 more minutes or until lentils are tender. Remove from heat. Remove and discard bay leaf.

3. Taste and adjust seasonings as desired before serving.

Variation: For an even heartier soup, add 2 chopped Savory Sausages (recipe in Chapter 12).

DEFINITION

Lacinato kale is an heirloom variety of kale that has tender, dark blue-green leaves and a slightly sweeter and more delicate taste than curly green kale. It's also referred to as Tuscan or Italian kale, or comically as dinosaur kale because the extremely wrinkled leaves have a somewhat prehistoric look.

Green and Gold Minestrone

Vegetable broth and nutritional yeast give the base of this hearty minestrone soup a nice golden color, and a generous assortment of green, yellow, and orange vegetables further enhances and complements this combination.

Yield:	Prep time:	Cook time:	Serving size:
2 quarts	15 to 20 minutes	40 to 45 minutes	1½ cups

6 cups water

2 cups low-sodium vegetable broth

1 cup Yukon gold potatoes, cut into quarters lengthwise and thinly sliced

⅔ cup carrots, cut into quarters lengthwise and thinly sliced

⅔ cup celery, cut in half lengthwise and thinly sliced

⅔ cup yellow onion, diced

⅔ cup yellow summer squash, cut into quarters lengthwise and thinly sliced

⅔ cup zucchini, cut into quarters lengthwise and thinly sliced

¼ cup Italian Herb Sprinkles (variation in Chapter 6) or nutritional yeast flakes

2 TB. garlic, minced

1 TB. Italian seasoning blend, or 1 tsp. each dried basil, oregano, and thyme

1 tsp. sea salt

½ tsp. freshly ground black pepper

½ tsp. crushed red pepper flakes

1 bay leaf

2 cups Swiss chard, roughly chopped and tightly packed

½ cup gluten-free ditalini, or other small-shape pasta

⅓ cup frozen peas

⅓ cup frozen shelled edamame

⅓ cup green onion, thinly sliced

⅓ cup chopped fresh parsley (preferably Italian flat-leaf)

1. In a large pot, combine water, vegetable broth, Yukon gold potatoes, carrots, celery, yellow onion, yellow summer squash, zucchini, Italian Herb Sprinkles, garlic, Italian seasoning blend, sea salt, pepper, crushed red pepper flakes, and bay leaf, and bring to a boil over high heat. Cover, reduce heat to low, and simmer for 30 minutes.

2. Add Swiss chard, ditalini, peas, edamame, green onion, and parsley, and cook for 10 to 12 more minutes or until pasta is al dente. Remove from heat. Remove and discard bay leaf.

3. Taste and adjust seasonings as desired before serving.

Variation: You can replace the Swiss chard with rainbow Swiss chard, baby spinach, or other greens.

CORNUCOPIA

Typically, only fresh pasta and egg noodles contain eggs because most dried pasta varieties are made only with a type of flour; water; a little salt; and depending on the variety, herbs, spices, and puréed vegetables or vegetable-based powders. So they're suitable for most vegans. Although most dried pasta is made with semolina flour or another wheat-based flour, you can find several varieties of gluten-free pasta right alongside the gluten-containing versions.

Apple and Butternut Bisque

If you're looking for a delicious and creamy fat-free soup, give this one a try. Made with apples, butternut squash purée, and spices, it's perfect for serving during the fall and winter months and at holiday gatherings.

Yield:	Prep time:	Cook time:	Serving size:
1½ quarts	7 to 10 minutes	15 to 20 minutes	1½ cups

1 cup yellow onion, diced

4½ cups water or low-sodium vegetable broth

2 large Fuji or Granny Smith apples, peeled, cored, and diced

2 TB. fresh ginger, minced

1 (15-oz.) can butternut squash purée

2 TB. maple syrup

1 tsp. ground cinnamon

¼ tsp. freshly grated nutmeg

Sea salt

Toasted sunflower seeds or pumpkin seeds

1. In a large pot, combine yellow onion and ½ cup water, and cook over medium heat, stirring often, for 3 minutes or until soft.

2. Add Fuji apples and ginger, and cook, stirring often, for 2 more minutes.

3. Stir in 2 cups water, and bring to a boil over high heat. Cover, reduce heat to low, and simmer for 5 to 7 minutes or until apples are soft. Remove from heat, and let cool slightly.

4. Transfer mixture to a blender or food processor fitted with an S blade, and process for 1 or 2 minutes or until smooth. Transfer the blended mixture back to the pot. (Alternatively, use an immersion blender and blend mixture directly in the pot until smooth.)

5. Stir in remaining 2 cups water, butternut squash purée, maple syrup, cinnamon, and nutmeg. Cover, reduce heat to low, and simmer for 5 minutes. Remove from heat, and season with sea salt as desired.

6. Top individual servings with toasted sunflower or pumpkin seeds as desired before serving.

Variation: You can replace the butternut squash purée with 1 (15-ounce) can sweet potato or pumpkin purée. For a lighter soup, whisk ¾ cup soy milk or other nondairy milk into the finished soup. For a spicier soup, replace the cinnamon and nutmeg with 1 teaspoon curry powder or chili powder.

CORNUCOPIA

Butternut squash and other winter squashes such as acorn, delicata, buttercup, turbans, and pumpkins are all high in vitamins A and C and are naturally sweet, so include them often in your meals during the fall and winter months. You can use them interchangeably for one another in recipes, and they're particularly delicious when roasted, steamed, or boiled.

Creamy California Vegetable Soup

During the winter months, there's nothing better for lunch or dinner than a big bowl of soup, and in less than an hour, you can enjoy this creamy, fat-free soup made with leeks, potatoes, frozen vegetables, and a bit of thyme and dill.

Yield:	Prep time:	Cook time:	Serving size:
2 quarts	15 minutes	25 minutes	1½ cups

3 cups water

1 (16-oz.) pkg. frozen California vegetable blend

1 leek, cut into quarters lengthwise and thinly sliced

2 cups red-skinned potatoes or Yukon gold potatoes, cut into quarters lengthwise and thinly sliced

1 cup low-sodium vegetable broth

2 TB. garlic, minced

2 TB. nutritional yeast flakes or Italian Herb Sprinkles (variation in Chapter 6)

1 TB. lemon juice

1½ tsp. dried thyme

1 tsp. sea salt

½ tsp. freshly ground black pepper

1½ cups soy milk or other nondairy milk

3 TB. cornstarch

⅓ cup chopped fresh parsley

2 TB. chopped fresh dill or 2 tsp. dried dill weed

1. In a large pot, combine water, California vegetable blend, leek, red-skinned potatoes, vegetable broth, garlic, nutritional yeast flakes, lemon juice, thyme, sea salt, and pepper, and bring to a boil over high heat. Cover, reduce heat to low, and simmer for 20 minutes.

2. In a small bowl, combine soy milk and cornstarch. Add soy milk mixture, parsley, and dill to the pot, and cook, stirring often, for 5 more minutes or until thickened. Remove from heat.

3. Taste and adjust seasonings as desired before serving.

Variation: If you like, replace the California vegetable blend with another variety of frozen vegetable blend, like Italian or mixed vegetables. You can bulk up this soup by adding 4 cups chopped kale or other greens.

MEATLESS AND WHEATLESS

Having a pantry and freezer well stocked with the items you most often use when cooking—like canned beans, tomato products, cartons of vegetable broth, roots, and assorted frozen vegetables—can really be a helping hand and time-saver for getting quick, yet healthy, meals on your table in no time.

Mexicali Chili

Colorful, spicy, chunky, and *caliente!* This chili is packed with peppers, onion, crushed tomatoes, several types of beans, a generous amount of spices, and chunks of our Beef-Style Gluten-Free Seitan for meatlike quality.

Yield:	Prep time:	Cook time:	Serving size:
2 quarts	10 to 15 minutes	20 minutes	1½ cups

1 cup yellow onion, diced

1 cup green bell pepper, diced

1 cup red bell pepper, diced

1 jalapeño pepper, ribs and seeds removed, and finely diced

2 TB. garlic, minced

1 TB. olive oil

2 cups water or low-sodium vegetable broth

1 (15-oz.) can mixed beans, drained and rinsed

1 (14-oz.) can fire-roasted crushed tomatoes

1 cup Beef-Style Gluten-Free Seitan (variation in Chapter 12), roughly chopped

2 tsp. cocoa powder

1½ tsp. sorghum syrup

1½ tsp. chili powder

1½ tsp. dried oregano

1 tsp. dried basil

1 tsp. ground cumin

½ tsp. sea salt

½ tsp. freshly ground black pepper

¼ tsp. cayenne or chipotle chili powder

⅓ cup chopped fresh cilantro

1 TB. lime juice

1. In a large pot, combine yellow onion, green bell pepper, red bell pepper, jalapeño pepper, garlic, and olive oil, and sauté over medium heat, stirring often, for 5 minutes.

2. Add water, mixed beans, crushed tomatoes, Beef-Style Gluten-Free Seitan, cocoa powder, sorghum syrup, chili powder, oregano, basil, cumin, sea salt, pepper, and cayenne, and stir well to combine. Increase heat to high, and bring to a boil.

3. Cover, reduce heat to low, and simmer for 15 minutes or until vegetables are tender. Remove from heat. Stir in cilantro and lime juice.

4. Taste and adjust seasonings as desired. Serve with tortilla chips, gluten-free crackers, or Country Cornbread (recipe in Chapter 5) as desired.

Variation: Feel free to replace the chopped gluten-free seitan with 1 (8-ounce) package tempeh, crumbled into small pieces with your fingers, or the mixed chili beans with 1 (15-ounce) can black, pinto, or kidney beans.

Plant-Based Dietitian Recommends: Omit the oil. Use ¼ cup water or vegetable broth in step 1 to sauté onions, peppers, and garlic, instead of using oil. Follow the rest of the directions by pouring the remaining liquid in during step 2.

MEATLESS AND WHEATLESS

Using mixed beans consisting of 2 or 3 different bean varieties combined all in one can in your recipes is a convenient way to include more types of beans into your diet, as well as an easy way to liven up your meals. In this chili recipe, we suggest using one that contains at least black, pinto, and kidney beans, but use whatever mixed bean blend appeals to you.

Thai Corn Chowder

In this Thai chowder, sweet corn is infused with sour *lemongrass* and lime, pungent ginger, earthy coriander, and spicy crushed red pepper flakes.

Yield:	Prep time:	Cook time:	Serving size:
2 quarts	10 minutes	20 to 25 minutes	1½ cups

2½ cups low-sodium vegetable broth or water

2 cups yellow onion, diced

2 large garlic cloves, minced

2 cups celery, diced

1 cup carrots, diced

1 cup red bell pepper, diced

1 TB. fresh ginger, minced

½ tsp. ground coriander

½ tsp. crushed red pepper flakes

4 cups frozen cut corn kernels, thawed

1 cup unsweetened coconut water

1 cup soy milk

2 TB. lemongrass, thinly sliced

⅓ cup chopped fresh cilantro

¼ cup lime juice

1 TB. lime zest

1. In a large pot, combine vegetable broth, yellow onion, and garlic, and sauté over medium heat, stirring often, for 3 minutes.

2. Add celery, carrots, and red bell pepper and sauté, stirring often, for 3 more minutes.

3. Add ginger, coriander, and crushed red pepper flakes, and sauté, stirring often, for 1 more minute.

4. Add 2 cups corn, coconut water, soy milk, and lemongrass, and bring to a boil over high heat. Cover, reduce heat to low, and simmer for 10 minutes. Remove from heat.

5. Using immersion blender, carefully blend chowder until smooth and creamy. Stir in remaining 2 cups corn, cilantro, lime juice, and lime zest. Place pot over medium-low heat, and simmer for 5 more minutes. Remove from heat, and serve hot.

Variation: If you don't have an immersion blender, you can carefully pour the chowder into a regular blender in batches instead. Return the blended chowder to the pot, and continue as directed.

> **DEFINITION**
>
> **Lemongrass** is a thick, lemon-scented grass commonly used in Thai dishes. When buying fresh lemongrass, look for stalks that are fragrant, tightly formed, and lemony-green. To prepare the stalks for use, remove the tough, outer leaves, and cut and discard the lower bulb. Then make thin slices up to ⅔ up the stalk. You can also use lemongrass that comes in a jar with water for easier preparation.

Sunday Dinner Stew

A hearty blend of tempeh, potatoes, pearl onions, carrots, celery, and peas, plus a bit of red wine, creates this one-pot meal that can feed a whole family of gluten-free vegans.

Yield:	Prep time:	Cook time:	Serving size:
2 quarts	8 to 10 minutes	25 to 30 minutes	1½ cups

3 cups low-sodium vegetable broth

2 cups red-skinned potatoes, cut into ½-in. cubes

1 (8-oz.) pkg. tempeh, cut into ½-in. cubes

1½ cups frozen pearl onions

1 cup carrots, sliced

1 cup celery, sliced

1½ TB. tomato paste

1½ TB. wheat-free tamari

1 tsp. garlic powder or garlic granules

¾ tsp. dried basil

¾ tsp. dried oregano

½ tsp. freshly ground black pepper or garlic pepper

½ cup frozen peas

2 TB. red wine

2 TB. chickpea/garbanzo bean flour or other gluten-free flour

2 TB. water

¼ cup chopped fresh parsley

1. In a large pot, combine vegetable broth, red-skinned potatoes, tempeh, pearl onions, carrots, celery, tomato paste, tamari, garlic powder, basil, oregano, and pepper, and bring to a boil over high heat. Cover, reduce heat to low, and simmer for 20 minutes or until vegetables are tender.

2. Stir in peas and red wine, and simmer for 2 more minutes.

3. In a small bowl, combine chickpea/garbanzo bean flour and water. Add to the pot, and cook, stirring often, for 3 to 5 more minutes or until thickened. Remove from heat and stir in parsley.

4. Taste and adjust seasonings as desired before serving hot with slices of Multi-Grain Sandwich Bread or Bettermilk Biscuits (recipes in Chapter 5).

Variation: Feel free to replace the tempeh cubes with cubes of Chicken-Style or Beef-Style Gluten-Free Seitan (recipe and variation in Chapter 12). You can also replace the potatoes with cubes of turnips, rutabagas, or parsnips.

> **CORNUCOPIA**
>
> Stews typically contain large chunks, cubes, or slices of vegetables and other ingredients, rather than small, diced pieces. Also, a stew has a much thicker consistency than your average soup because it's almost always thickened with a slurry mixture, made by combining either flour or a starch with water or other liquid.

Exceptional Entrées and Side Dishes

In Part 5, we've assembled some of our favorite recipes for the main meal of the day. Forget the take-out menu. In the mood for pasta, pizza, a burrito, or curry? It's all in Part 5. Need to feed a family of four easily and on a budget? You'll find many cost-effective casseroles and amply portioned options in the following recipes.

To balance out the entrées on your dinner plate, we've included a whole slew of grain-, bean-, and veggie-based side dishes. Or if you prefer, you can combine them as your hunger dictates to create your own DIY dinner.

And once you've managed to make these dishes your own, feel free to host your own themed dinner party or holiday shindig so you can show your friends and family how gourmet gluten-free vegan cooking can be!

Plentiful Pasta

In This Chapter

- Raw veggie pastas
- International noodle dishes
- Oven-baked casseroles for a crowd

We bet when you first went gluten free, one of your first thoughts was *Oh no! No more bread and pasta for me!* Well, that just isn't so. In Chapter 5, we provided recipes for making your own breads, both sweet and sandwich-style, and even a batch of biscuits and hamburger buns. In this chapter, we introduce you to some of our favorite ways to prepare gluten-free pasta! Yes, we said *pasta!*

Wheat and semolina aren't the only suitable flours for making pasta; other tasty varieties are made from white and brown rice, buckwheat, corn, quinoa, or a combination of gluten-free grains. Some of our favorite brands are Ancient Harvest, Bionaturae, DeBoles, Glutino, Orgran, and Tinkyada, so give them a try and see which ones suit your taste buds best.

In this chapter, we have recipes for noodles Asian-style or tossed with cooked veggies or bitter greens, as well as a creamy Mac 'n' Cheese and baked lasagna. And for some super-healthy "pasta," we show you how to turn fresh veggies into strandlike stand-ins. *Buon appetito* (Italian for "have a good meal")!

Raw Zucchini Noodles with Pesto

Here, humble zucchini and other vegetables are transformed into a plate of pasta topped with a flavorful pesto sauce.

Yield:	Prep time:	Serving size:
4 cups	8 to 10 minutes	1 to 1¼ cups

2 large zucchini

1 large Roma tomato, diced

¼ cup Basil, Spinach, and Pumpkin Seed Pesto (recipe in Chapter 9)

¼ cup water

½ tsp. crushed red pepper flakes

Himalayan pink salt or sea salt

Freshly ground black pepper

1 TB. raw pine nuts or hemp seeds

1. To make zucchini noodles, use a *spiralizer* to make long spaghetti- or fettuccine-style strands. (Alternatively, cut each zucchini in half lengthwise. Make a V-shape cut to remove most of the seed section, and slice the removed seed section into thin, long strips with a knife. Use a vegetable peeler to shave long strips down the entire length of each zucchini half.)

2. Transfer zucchini noodles to a medium bowl. Add Roma tomato; Basil, Spinach, and Pumpkin Seed Pesto; water; and crushed red pepper flakes, and toss gently to evenly coat noodles.

3. Taste and season with Himalayan pink salt and pepper as desired. Sprinkle pine nuts over top, and serve immediately.

Variation: For an even more colorful noodle dish, make the noodles using 2 medium carrots, 1 yellow summer squash, and 1 medium zucchini instead.

DEFINITION

Spiralizer (a.k.a. spiral slicer) is a kitchen gadget that quickly and easily creates spiral strands, curly ribbons, or paper-thin slices of fruits and vegetables. Place the item onto the spiralizer's prongs and turn the handle while pushing the base toward the blade to make continuous spiral strands. Find them in kitchen supply stores and online.

Szechuan Noodles

In this Asian-style noodle dish, pineapple juice, tamari, brown rice syrup, and vinegar combine with a generous dose of garlic, ginger, and crushed red pepper flakes to create a sweet-and-sour sauce, perfect for coating strands of brown rice spaghetti.

Yield:	Prep time:	Cook time:	Serving size:
8 cups	10 to 20 minutes	18 to 20 minutes (depending on pasta variety)	1½ cups

1 (12-oz.) pkg. brown rice spaghetti or other gluten-free spaghetti

⅔ cup pineapple juice

⅓ cup wheat-free tamari or Bragg Liquid Aminos

⅓ cup brown rice vinegar

2 TB. toasted sesame oil

2 TB. gluten-free brown rice syrup

2 TB. garlic, minced

2 TB. fresh ginger, minced

1 tsp. crushed red pepper flakes

½ tsp. freshly ground black pepper

1 cup carrots, shredded

½ cup green onion, thinly sliced

½ cup chopped fresh cilantro

¼ cup chopped fresh parsley

2 TB. *gomasio,* sesame seeds, or black sesame seeds

1. Fill a large saucepan ⅔ full of water, and bring to a boil over medium-high heat. Add brown rice spaghetti, and cook, stirring occasionally, according to the package directions or until al dente. Remove from heat. Drain spaghetti in a colander, but do not rinse. Transfer hot spaghetti to a large bowl.

2. Meanwhile, in a small glass bowl, whisk together pineapple juice, tamari, brown rice vinegar, toasted sesame oil, brown rice syrup, garlic, ginger, crushed red pepper flakes, and pepper.

3. Pour pineapple juice mixture over brown rice spaghetti, and using a pair of tongs, toss well to evenly coat spaghetti. Set aside for 5 to 10 minutes or until all liquid is absorbed.

4. Add carrots, green onion, cilantro, parsley, and gomasio, and toss well to combine. Serve hot, cold, or at room temperature as desired.

Variation: Feel free to add 1 cup roughly chopped Miso-Glazed Tofu (recipe in Chapter 12). For **Veggie Lo Mein,** use only ½ cup shredded carrots, and add ½ cup fresh or thawed frozen pea pods, cut in half diagonally, ½ cup each shredded napa and red cabbages, ½ cup diced red bell pepper, ½ cup Fresh and Flavorful Sprouts using mung beans (recipe in Chapter 10), and ¼ cup roughly chopped toasted peanuts or cashews.

Plant-Based Dietitian Recommends: Omit the oil.

> **DEFINITION**
>
> Made from dry-roasted sesame seeds that have been ground together with a little sea salt, **gomasio** can be used as a condiment on noodles, rice and other cooked grains, miso soup, stir-fries, and other Asian dishes in place of sesame seeds. It's also a tasty seasoning that can replace table salt.

Buckwheat Noodle Bowls

When you're in the mood for something warm and cozy, this dish is for you. Buckwheat provides a unique flavor that nicely complements the classic tangy miso. Salty, pungent, and hearty, this souplike bowl will satisfy.

Yield:	Prep time:	Cook time:	Serving size:
8 cups	10 to 20 minutes	20 to 25 minutes	1½ cups

1 (8-oz.) pkg. 100 percent whole buckwheat soba noodles

2 cups leeks, finely chopped

1 TB. garlic, minced

4 cups low-sodium vegetable broth

1 TB. fresh or jarred ginger, minced

¼ cup wheat-free tamari or Bragg Liquid Aminos

¼ cup brown rice vinegar

2 cups shiitake or crimini mushrooms, thinly sliced

2 cups water

4 cups bok choy, coarsely chopped

¼ cup mellow miso

½ cup chopped fresh cilantro

2 TB. gomasio, sesame seeds, or black sesame seeds

1. Fill a medium saucepan ⅔ full of water, and bring to a boil over medium-high heat. Add buckwheat soba noodles, and cook, stirring occasionally, for 6 to 8 minutes or according to the package directions. Remove from heat. Drain

noodles in a colander, but do not rinse. Transfer hot buckwheat noodles to a medium bowl.

2. In a large soup pot over medium heat, sauté leeks and garlic in 1 cup vegetable broth, stirring often, for 5 minutes or until leeks are soft. Add ginger, tamari, brown rice vinegar, mushrooms, and water, and cook, stirring often, for 5 more minutes.

3. Add remaining 3 cups vegetable broth, increase heat to medium-high, and bring to a boil. Add bok choy and buckwheat noodles, reduce heat to low, separate noodles with tongs to avoid sticking, and simmer for 2 to 4 more minutes or until bok choy is wilted.

4. In a small bowl, stir together mellow miso with 6 tablespoons broth from the soup pot until dissolved. Remove soup pot from heat, and stir in miso mixture and cilantro leaves. Top individual servings with a light sprinkle of gomasio as desired, and serve hot.

Variation: Feel free to add 1 cup chopped tofu or vegetables like 1 cup chopped broccoli, shredded carrots, or chopped kale.

AGAINST THE GRAIN

Buckwheat, despite the name, is unrelated to wheat. Instead, it's a gluten-free pseudocereal (broadleaf nongrass plants used in similar ways as cereals such as amaranth, quinoa, and buckwheat) that can be used as a whole grain or made into noodles. Buckwheat is high in fiber, tryptophan, and manganese. When selecting soba noodles, be certain to choose 100 percent buckwheat because most so-called buckwheat noodles are combined with whole wheat.

Spinach Spaghetti with Tomatoes and Pumpkin Seeds

Latin flavors come alive in this vibrant pasta dish featuring spinach-flavored spaghetti tossed with fresh tomatoes and bell peppers, salty black olives, fragrant cilantro, and freshly toasted pumpkin seeds.

Yield:	Prep time:	Cook time:	Serving size:
9 cups	15 to 20 minutes	15 to 20 minutes (depending on pasta variety)	1½ cups

1 (12-oz.) pkg. brown rice spinach spaghetti or other gluten-free spaghetti

½ cup raw pumpkin seeds

1 cup red onion, diced

⅔ cup green bell pepper, diced

⅔ cup red bell pepper, diced

1 jalapeño pepper, ribs and seeds removed, and finely diced

1½ TB. olive oil

3 cups Roma tomatoes or assorted heirloom tomatoes, diced

2 TB. garlic, minced

2 tsp. dried oregano

2 tsp. chili powder

1 tsp. smoked paprika

¾ tsp. sea salt

½ tsp. freshly ground black pepper

½ tsp. crushed red pepper flakes or chipotle chili powder

½ cup low-sodium vegetable broth

½ cup chopped fresh cilantro

¼ cup kalamata olives or other black olives, pitted and roughly chopped

2½ TB. Spicy Sprinkles (recipe in Chapter 6) or nutritional yeast flakes

1. Fill a large saucepan ⅔ full of water, and bring to a boil over medium-high heat. Add brown rice spinach spaghetti, and cook, stirring occasionally, according to the package directions or until al dente. Remove from heat. Drain spaghetti in a colander, but do not rinse.

2. Meanwhile, in a small, nonstick skillet, place pumpkin seeds, and cook over medium heat, shaking saucepan often, for 3 to 5 minutes or until lightly toasted and fragrant. Transfer pumpkin seeds to a small bowl, and set aside.

3. Place a large, nonstick skillet over medium heat. Add red onion, green bell pepper, red bell pepper, jalapeño pepper, and olive oil, and sauté, stirring often, for 7 minutes.

4. Add Roma tomatoes, garlic, oregano, chili powder, smoked paprika, sea salt, pepper, and crushed red pepper flakes, and cook, stirring often, for 3 to 5 more minutes or until vegetables are tender. Remove from heat.

5. Add hot spinach spaghetti, vegetable broth, cilantro, kalamata olives, and Spicy Sprinkles to the skillet. Using a pair of tongs, toss well to combine. Top individual servings with additional Spicy Sprinkles as desired, and serve hot.

Variation: Feel free to replace the spinach spaghetti with fettuccine or other gluten-free pasta shape. For **Fiesta Spaghetti,** add to the sautéed vegetable mixture $\frac{1}{2}$ cup each yellow summer squash and zucchini, cut into quarters lengthwise and thinly sliced, $\frac{1}{2}$ cup fresh or frozen cut corn kernels. When adding the cooked spaghetti, throw in $\frac{1}{2}$ cup canned black or red beans.

Plant-Based Dietitian Recommends: Instead of the olive oil, you can substitute $\frac{1}{2}$ cup vegetable broth or water.

CORNUCOPIA

Pumpkin seeds are sometimes referred to by their Spanish name, *pepitas*. Even though they're actually the same thing, most often pepitas are sold with their outer protective hulls (or shells) removed, while pumpkin seeds are sold both ways, as well as raw, or roasted with or without salt or other seasonings. When we call for pumpkin seeds in these recipes, we mean the plain, shelled variety.

Penne with Tempeh Italiano and Broccoli Rabe

Penne pasta holds its own, complementing the bold flavors of our spicy Tempeh Italiano and slightly bitter broccoli rabe, and our Spicy Sprinkles provide a Parmesan-like final finish.

Yield:	Prep time:	Cook time:	Serving size:
8 or 9 cups	15 minutes	10 to 12 minutes (depending on pasta variety)	1½ cups

1 (8-oz.) pkg. corn or brown rice penne, or other gluten-free shaped pasta

½ cup yellow onion, diced

1½ TB. garlic, minced

½ TB. olive oil

1 medium bunch broccoli rabe (about 1½ lb.), cut into rough 1-in. pieces

½ cup low-sodium vegetable broth or water

1 cup Tempeh Italiano (recipe in Chapter 12)

⅓ cup fresh basil, cut chiffonade, or chopped fresh parsley (preferably Italian flat-leaf parsley)

2 TB. Spicy Sprinkles (recipe in Chapter 6) or nutritional yeast flakes

½ tsp. crushed red pepper flakes

Sea salt

Freshly ground black pepper

1. Fill a large saucepan ⅔ full of water, and bring to a boil over medium-high heat. Add corn penne, and cook, stirring occasionally, according to the package directions or until al dente. Remove from heat. Drain penne in a colander, but do not rinse.

2. Meanwhile, place a large nonstick skillet over medium heat. Add yellow onion, garlic, and olive oil, and sauté, stirring often, for 3 minutes.

3. Add broccoli rabe and vegetable broth, and cook, stirring often, for 3 to 5 more minutes or until broccoli rabe is crisp-tender. Add Tempeh Italiano, and cook, stirring often, for 1 more minute. Remove from heat.

4. Add hot penne, basil, Spicy Sprinkles, and crushed red pepper flakes, and stir well to combine. Taste and season with sea salt and pepper as desired. Top individual servings with additional Spicy Sprinkles as desired, and serve hot.

Variation: Feel free to replace the penne with fusilli, rigatoni, or ziti.

Plant-Based Dietitian Recommends: Substitute ¼ cup vegetable broth or water for the olive oil.

CORNUCOPIA

Broccoli rabe (a.k.a. rapini) is a member of the brassica family and has bitter-tasting spiked leaves with small green florets that look quite similar to broccoli florets. It's usually in the produce section of most grocery stores, but if you can't find it, you can replace it in this recipe with 1 cup small broccoli florets and 4 cups roughly chopped Swiss chard, lacinato kale, or spinach.

Baked Rainbow Rigatoni Casserole

This hearty Italian-style dish features gluten-free rigatoni, a vibrant assortment of cooked vegetables, rainbow Swiss chard, and creamy tofu ricotta, all covered with marinara sauce and vegan cheese.

Yield:	Prep time:	Cook time:	Serving size:
10 to 12 cups (depending on pasta variety)	20 to 30 minutes	40 to 45 minutes (depending on pasta variety)	1½ cups

1 (1-lb.) pkg. gluten-free rigatoni

⅓ cup carrots, finely diced

⅓ cup red onion, finely diced

⅓ cup green bell pepper, diced

⅓ cup red bell pepper, diced

⅓ cup low-sodium vegetable broth or water

½ cup fresh or frozen broccoli florets, roughly chopped

⅓ cup yellow summer squash, diced

⅓ cup zucchini, diced

2 TB. garlic, minced

½ tsp. dried oregano

½ tsp. freshly ground black pepper

2½ cups Tofu Ricotta (recipe in Chapter 6)

¼ cup fresh basil, cut chiffonade

¼ cup chopped fresh parsley (preferably Italian flat-leaf parsley)

2 TB. Italian Herb Sprinkles (variation in Chapter 6) or Spicy Sprinkles (recipe in Chapter 6) or nutritional yeast flakes

3 cups rainbow Swiss chard or red Swiss chard, stems thinly sliced and leaves cut chiffonade

3½ cups Five-Minute Marinara (recipe in Chapter 9)

1 cup shredded Mellow Jack Cheese (recipe in Chapter 6)

1. Fill a large saucepan ⅔ full of water, and bring to a boil over medium-high heat. Add rigatoni, and cook, stirring occasionally, according to the package directions or until al dente. Remove from heat. Drain rigatoni in a colander, but do not rinse.

2. Meanwhile, place a large, nonstick skillet over medium heat. Add carrots, red onion, green bell pepper, red bell pepper, and vegetable broth, and cook, stirring often, for 5 minutes.

3. Add broccoli, yellow summer squash, zucchini, garlic, oregano, and pepper, and cook, stirring often, for 3 minutes. Remove from heat.

4. Preheat the oven to 375°F. Lightly oil a 9×13-inch baking pan or large casserole dish.

5. Transfer cooked rigatoni to a large bowl. Add Tofu Ricotta, basil, parsley, and 1 tablespoon Italian Herb Sprinkles, and stir well to evenly coat rigatoni. Add cooked vegetable mixture and rainbow Swiss chard, and stir well to combine.

6. Transfer rigatoni mixture to the prepared baking pan. Top with Five-Minute Marinara, and sprinkle shredded Mellow Jack Cheese and remaining 1 table-spoon Italian Herb Sprinkles over top.

7. Bake for 30 minutes or until heated through and lightly browned around edges. Remove from the oven. Top individual servings with additional Italian Herb Sprinkles as desired, and serve hot.

Variation: Penne or ziti work well as substitutes for the rigatoni, and Cashew Ricotta (variation in Chapter 6) is a suitable replacement for the Tofu Ricotta. To adapt this recipe to make **Stuffed Shells,** cook the shells according to the package instructions. Stir together the Tofu Ricotta, cooked vegetables, rainbow Swiss chard, and 1 tablespoon Italian Herb Sprinkles, and use this mixture to fill the cooked shells. Then, top them with Five-Minute Marinara sauce and Mellow Jack Cheese, and bake as directed.

MEATLESS AND WHEATLESS

Tinkyada makes some of the best-tasting rice-based, gluten-free pastas, and they're available in 18 different shapes and flavor varieties, such as white or brown rice, spinach, and mixed vegetable. Not only do they offer spaghetti, fettuccine, elbows, spirals, and such, but they also sell lasagna noodles and grand shells.

White Lasagna with Spinach and Chanterelle Mushrooms

An elegant and impressive lasagna is made with alternating layers of brown rice noodles, Tofu Ricotta, fresh spinach, and lightly sautéed and white wine–infused chanterelle mushrooms and onion.

Yield:	Prep time:	Cook time:	Serving size:
1 (9×13-inch) pan or 12 pieces	15 to 20 minutes (depending on spinach used)	50 to 60 minutes	1 piece

1½ lb. chanterelle mushrooms or a mixture of other mushrooms, cut in half and thinly sliced

⅔ cup yellow onion or shallots, diced

½ TB. olive oil

1½ TB. garlic, minced

½ tsp. sea salt

½ tsp. freshly ground black pepper or garlic pepper

⅓ cup white wine

4 cups hot Béchamel Sauce (recipe in Chapter 9) or Lite White Sauce (variation in Chapter 9)

1½ cups Mellow Jack Cheese (recipe in Chapter 6), shredded

¼ cup plus 1 TB. nutritional yeast flakes

1 (10-oz.) pkg. brown rice lasagna noodles or other gluten-free lasagna noodles

2½ cups Tofu Ricotta (recipe in Chapter 6)

2 (5-oz.) pkg. baby spinach, or 2 bunches spinach, triple washed, stems removed, and torn into bite-size pieces

1. Place a large, nonstick skillet over medium heat. Add chanterelle mushrooms, yellow onion, and olive oil, and sauté, stirring often, for 5 minutes or until vegetables are soft.

2. Add garlic, sea salt, and pepper, and sauté, stirring often, for 2 more minutes. Add white wine, and cook, stirring often, for 1 more minute. Remove from heat.

3. Preheat the oven to 375°F. Lightly oil a 9×13-inch baking pan or large casserole dish.

4. In a large bowl, combine hot Béchamel Sauce, ½ cup shredded Mellow Jack Cheese, and ¼ cup nutritional yeast flakes.

5. To assemble lasagna, spoon ¾ cup Béchamel Sauce into the bottom of the prepared baking pan. Place 3 uncooked lasagna noodles side by side on top of Béchamel Sauce, top with ⅓ of Tofu Ricotta, ⅓ of baby spinach, ⅓ of chanterelle mushroom mixture, and top with 1 cup Béchamel Sauce. Repeat layering procedure 2 more times.

6. Place last 3 uncooked lasagna noodles side by side on top, followed by remaining Béchamel Sauce, and sprinkle remaining 1 cup shredded Mellow Jack Cheese and remaining 1 tablespoon nutritional yeast flakes over top.

7. Cover baking pan with a lid or a layer of parchment paper and aluminum foil, and bake for 35 minutes. Remove the lid and bake for 5 to 10 more minutes or until lightly browned on top. Remove from the oven. Top individual servings with additional nutritional yeast flakes as desired, and serve hot.

Variation: Feel free to replace the Tofu Ricotta with Cashew Ricotta (variation in Chapter 6). For added flavor and color, add 1 diced medium red bell pepper or 1 cup sun-dried tomato pieces to the sautéed chanterelle mushroom mixture.

Plant-Based Dietitian Recommends: Substitute ¼ cup vegetable broth or water for the olive oil. Use silicone bakeware to avoid sticking.

CORNUCOPIA

You don't need to precook the lasagna noodles if your lasagna contains enough ingredients with a high water (or moisture) content, like the fresh spinach used in this recipe. As the lasagna cooks, the spinach will wilt and release enough moisture to soften the noodles. The Béchamel Sauce will add moisture, too. Also, covering your lasagna with a lid (or parchment paper and aluminum foil) creates some steam inside the pan, which also helps soften the noodles.

Mac 'n' Cheese

We've given the classic American comfort food a gluten-free vegan makeover by using plump corn and quinoa elbows, mixed with our Cheesy Sauce and shredded Mellow Jack Cheese—or Better Cheddar if you prefer a more robust flavor!

Yield:	Prep time:	Cook time:	Serving size:
5 cups	8 to 10 minutes	10 minutes (depending on pasta variety)	1¼ cups

1 (8-oz.) pkg. corn and quinoa elbows or other gluten-free shaped pasta

1½ cups hot Cheesy Sauce (recipe in Chapter 6)

¾ cup Mellow Jack Cheese or Better Cheddar (recipes in Chapter 6), shredded

½ cup soy milk or other nondairy milk

¼ tsp. sea salt

¼ tsp. freshly ground black pepper

1. Fill a large saucepan ⅔ full of water, and bring to a boil over medium-high heat. Add elbows, and cook, stirring occasionally, according to the package directions or until al dente. Remove from heat. Drain elbows in a colander, but do not rinse.

2. In a large bowl, combine hot Cheesy Sauce, shredded Mellow Jack Cheese, soy milk, sea salt, and pepper. Add hot elbows, and stir gently to combine. Serve hot.

Variation: You can also prepare this Mac 'n' Cheese by combining the cooked elbows with 2 cups hot Béchamel Sauce (recipe in Chapter 9), 1 cup shredded Mellow Jack Cheese (or Better Cheddar), sea salt, and pepper. For a bit of color, add 1 cup frozen and thawed broccoli florets or ½ cup peas to the hot Mac 'n' Cheese.

MEATLESS AND WHEATLESS

Typically, when mentioning mac 'n' cheese, the average American envisions the yellow-orange concoction prepared using a packaged box and its powdered seasoning mixture. To easily replicate a similar hue in our gluten-free vegan version, we use golden, yellow-colored corn and quinoa elbows.

Veggie All-Stars

In This Chapter

- Spicy and savory curries and paneer
- Gluten-free pizza
- Enticing rolls and layered entrées

As a vegan, you likely eat a wide variety of plant-based foods such as beans and legumes, grains, leafy greens, and veggies of all shapes, sizes, and textures to fill your protein quota. Although some of the recipes in this chapter do contain tofu or some of our gluten-free seitan specialties, vegetables are the star attraction of the entrées in this chapter.

We both like to dabble in different ethnic and regional cuisine varieties, so we've also included a collection of recipes from here to across the globe. If you're craving Mexican or Latin food, Indian cuisine, or even pizza, we've got you covered.

You'll also learn how truly easy it can be to "veganize" some classic oven-baked casseroles, all of which employ several recipes from other chapters in this book and are guaranteed to satisfy even the heartiest of appetites—gluten free and vegan or not. So get ready to tie one on—an apron, that is!—because we're serving up dinner gluten-free vegan style!

Rice and Bean Burrito Supreme

These *grande* vegan beauties are filled with the works—layers of seasoned rice and bean filling, shredded lettuce, our homemade vegan cheese, spicy guacamole, salsa, and tofu sour cream.

Yield:	Prep time:	Cook time:	Serving size:
6 burritos	10 to 12 minutes	5 to 7 minutes	1 burrito

⅓ cup green onion, thinly sliced

¼ cup water or low-sodium vegetable broth

1 jalapeño pepper, ribs and seeds removed, and finely diced

1 TB. garlic, minced

½ tsp. chili powder

½ tsp. dried oregano

¼ tsp. ground cumin

1 cup cooked short-grain brown rice or other rice

1 cup canned red beans or other beans, drained and rinsed

¼ cup chopped fresh cilantro

Sea salt

Freshly ground black pepper

6 (8-in.) brown rice, hemp, or other gluten-free tortillas

2 cups shredded loose-leaf lettuce or other lettuce

Shredded Better Cheddar or Mellow Jack Cheese (recipes in Chapter 6)

Whoo-Pea Guacamole (recipe in Chapter 8), or 1 medium Hass avocado, peeled, pitted, and diced

Tofu Sour Cream (recipe in Chapter 9)

Sausalito Salsa (recipe in Chapter 8) or store-bought salsa

1. Place a medium, nonstick skillet over medium heat. Add green onion, water, jalapeño pepper, and garlic, and cook, stirring often, for 2 minutes.

2. Add chili powder, oregano, and cumin, and cook, stirring often, for 1 more minute. Add brown rice, red beans, and cilantro, and cook, stirring often, for 1 or 2 more minutes or until rice and beans are heated through. Remove from heat. Taste and season with sea salt and pepper as desired.

3. For easier rolling, warm each tortilla in a large skillet over medium heat for 1 or 2 minutes per side. Alternatively, warm tortillas in the microwave for 20 to 30 seconds.

4. To assemble each burrito, place 1 warmed tortilla flat on a large cutting board or work surface. Place $\frac{1}{3}$ cup shredded lettuce horizontally in center of tortilla. Spoon $\frac{1}{3}$ cup rice mixture on top of lettuce. On top, layer, in order, shredded Better Cheddar, Whoo-Pea Guacamole, Tofu Sour Cream, and Sausalito Salsa as desired.

5. To finish rolling each burrito, fold bottom half of tortilla over filling, fold in each side toward the center over filling, and roll up from bottom edge to enclose filling. Place burrito seam side down on a plate.

6. Repeat assembly and rolling procedure with remaining tortillas, rice mixture, and other filling ingredients. Serve immediately.

Variation: You can omit the canned red beans and replace them with heated vegetarian refried beans. For **Wet Burritos,** leave out the shredded lettuce and Whoo-Pea Guacamole, and place rolled burritos seam side down on plates. Spoon a $\frac{1}{4}$ cup hot Cheesy Sauce (recipe in Chapter 6) and 2 or 3 tablespoons Roasted Tomatillo and Avocado Salsa or Sausalito Salsa (recipes in Chapter 8) over each burrito—or use both! Garnish with shredded lettuce, and serve Whoo-Pea Guacamole and Tofu Sour Cream on the side.

AGAINST THE GRAIN

When purchasing tortillas, check the label to be sure they're gluten free and vegan because many manufacturers use honey as a sweetener. Also closely look at the fat content of each tortilla. Although they seem like a healthy option, you may be surprised to see how the fat content differs from brand to brand.

Cabbage Rolls

We've veganized this family favorite by omitting the meat and replacing it with our Savory Sausages and adding a blend of sautéed and seasoned vegetables, brown rice, and some marinara sauce.

Yield:	Prep time:	Cook time:	Serving size:
12 to 14 cabbage rolls	20 to 25 minutes	45 to 55 minutes	2 cabbage rolls

1 large head cabbage, core removed

1½ cups yellow onion, diced

1½ cups celery, diced

1 cup green bell pepper, diced

1 cup red bell pepper, diced

½ TB. olive oil

2 Savory Sausages (recipe in Chapter 12), cut into quarters lengthwise, and thinly sliced, or 2 cups Beef-Style Gluten-Free Seitan, roughly chopped (variation in Chapter 12)

1½ TB. garlic, minced

1½ TB. Italian seasoning blend or 1½ tsp. each dried basil, oregano, and thyme

¾ tsp. sea salt

½ tsp. freshly ground black pepper

3½ cups hot Five-Minute Marinara (recipe in Chapter 9)

1 cup low-sodium vegetable broth or water

3 cups cooked long- or short-grain brown rice

1½ TB. Spicy Sprinkles (recipe in Chapter 6) or nutritional yeast flakes

1. Fill a large soup pot ⅔ full of water, and bring to a boil over medium-high heat. Carefully place head of cabbage in boiling water, and cook for 10 minutes. Remove from heat. Immerse head of cabbage into a large bowl of cold water, and set aside for 5 minutes.

2. Preheat the oven to 350°F. Lightly oil a 9×13-inch baking pan or large casserole dish, or use a silicone baking pan.

3. While cabbage is cooking, place a large, nonstick skillet over medium heat. Add yellow onion, celery, green bell pepper, red bell pepper, and olive oil, and sauté, stirring often, for 5 minutes.

4. Add Savory Sausages, garlic, Italian seasoning blend, sea salt, and pepper, and sauté, stirring often, for 3 to 5 more minutes or until vegetables are soft. Remove from heat.

5. When head of cabbage is cool enough to handle, remove large outer leaves (at least 12 to 14 leaves), and place them on a large plate. Roughly chop remaining cabbage, and set aside.

6. In a small bowl, combine $1\frac{1}{2}$ cups Five-Minute Marinara and vegetable broth, and set aside.

7. In a large bowl, combine remaining 2 cups Five-Minute Marinara, cooked vegetable mixture, reserved chopped cabbage, brown rice, and Spicy Sprinkles.

8. Place 1 cabbage leaf on a large plate or work surface. Place $\frac{1}{2}$ cup filling mixture at core end of cabbage leaf, fold in each side of leaf toward the center over filling, and roll up from core end of cabbage leaf to enclose filling. Place cabbage roll seam side down in the prepared baking pan. Repeat assembly and rolling procedure for remaining cabbage leaves and filling mixture.

9. Pour reserved marinara-broth mixture over top of cabbage rolls. Cover the baking pan with a lid or a layer of parchment paper and aluminum foil, and bake for 30 to 35 minutes. Remove from the oven. Serve hot, 2 cabbage rolls per person.

Variation: Large collard greens or Swiss chard leaves are a good stand-in for the cabbage leaves, and the brown rice can be replaced with an equal amount of other cooked grains such as quinoa or millet. To use the rice-vegetable filling mixture to make a batch of **Stuffed Peppers,** cut 6 large bell peppers in half lengthwise, and remove the stems, ribs, and seeds. Fill each pepper half with $\frac{1}{2}$ cup filling, place them side by side in a baking pan, cover with the marinara-broth mixture, and bake as directed or until peppers are tender.

Plant-Based Dietitian Recommends: Use silicone bakeware instead of the oiled baking pan, and substitute $\frac{1}{2}$ cup vegetable broth or water for the oil. Add more liquid if necessary while sautéing.

CORNUCOPIA

Beans, broccoli, brussels sprouts, cauliflower, and cabbage contain an indigestible carbohydrate known as raffinose that can cause flatulence and bloating for some people. If eating these foods causes you discomfort, avoid them or eat them in smaller, but more consistent, doses to help reduce these symptoms.

Mattar Tofu Paneer

In our vegan version of the popular Indian mattar paneer masala, tofu cubes that have been baked and simmered in a spicy sauce flavored with spices, ground nuts, tomatoes, vegan yogurt, and peas are a perfect stand-in for paneer cheese.

Yield:	Prep time:	Cook time:	Serving size:
6 cups	15 minutes	35 to 40 minutes	1 cup

1 TB. *garam masala*

2 tsp. curry powder

1 tsp. ground coriander

1 tsp. ground cumin

1 tsp. smoked paprika or chili powder

1 tsp. onion powder

1 tsp. garlic powder or garlic granules

1 lb. firm or extra-firm tofu, cut into $\frac{1}{2}$-in. cubes

1$\frac{1}{2}$ TB. olive oil

2 tsp. nutritional yeast flakes

6 TB. unsalted roasted peanuts or raw cashews

1 cup unsweetened coconut water

$\frac{1}{2}$ cup plain vegan yogurt

1 cup yellow onion, finely diced

1 jalapeño pepper, ribs and seeds removed, and finely diced

2 TB. garlic, minced

2 TB. fresh ginger, minced

3 cups tomatoes, finely diced

1 tsp. sea salt

1 cup fresh or frozen peas

$\frac{2}{3}$ cup chopped fresh cilantro

1 TB. lime juice

1. In a small bowl, combine garam masala, curry powder, coriander, cumin, smoked paprika, onion powder, and garlic powder, and set aside.

2. Preheat the oven to 425°F. Line a large cookie sheet with parchment paper or a Silpat liner.

3. Place tofu cubes on the prepared cookie sheet. Drizzle 1 tablespoon olive oil evenly over tofu cubes, and sprinkle $\frac{1}{2}$ of garam masala mixture and nutritional yeast flakes over top. Using your hands, gently toss tofu cubes until evenly coated, and spread them out into a single layer.

4. Bake for 15 minutes. Remove from the oven. Stir tofu cubes with a spatula, and spread them out into a single layer again. Bake for 10 to 15 more minutes or until tofu cubes are slightly firm and lightly browned around the edges. Remove from the oven.

5. While tofu cubes are baking, prepare masala sauce. In a food processor fitted with an S blade, place roasted peanuts, and process for 1 minute or until a fine powder. Transfer to a small bowl, stir in coconut water and yogurt, and set aside.

6. Place a large, nonstick skillet over medium heat. Add yellow onion, jalapeño pepper, garlic, ginger, remaining garam masala mixture, and remaining $\frac{1}{2}$ tablespoon olive oil, and sauté, stirring often, for 3 minutes.

7. Add tomatoes and sea salt, and sauté, stirring often, for 7 to 10 more minutes or until tomatoes are soft.

8. Reduce heat to low, stir in yogurt mixture and peas, and simmer, stirring often, for 3 minutes. Add tofu cubes, and simmer, stirring often, for 2 more minutes. Remove from heat. Stir in cilantro and lime juice, and serve hot over cooked brown rice or other grains as desired.

Variation: For added texture and a heartier dish, add 1 cup cauliflower florets and 1 cup potatoes, cut into $\frac{1}{2}$-inch cubes, to the sautéing onion mixture.

Plant-Based Dietitian Recommends: Substitute 2 tablespoons coconut water, vegetable broth, or water for the olive oil drizzled on the tofu and an additional $\frac{1}{4}$ cup of the same liquid for sautéing.

> **DEFINITION**
>
> *Garam masala* in Hindi literally means "hot spice." Although it's made with a blend of pungent and warming spices, it doesn't necessarily have a hot flavor like cayenne or chili powder. This flavorful blend is commonly used in Indian and Southern Asian cuisines as an alternative to curry powder. Blends vary by brand, but most contain cardamom, cinnamon, coriander, cumin, cloves, and black pepper.

Indian Green Curry

Curries are spicy, savory stews that originated and reign supreme in India; this spicy all-vegetable version is aptly named for the assorted green vegetables it contains.

Yield:	Prep time:	Cook time:	Serving size:
6 servings	10 to 15 minutes	25 to 35 minutes	1¼ cups

3 cups Yukon gold potatoes, cut into 1-in. cubes

2 cups cauliflower, cut into small florets

1 cup yellow onion, diced

½ TB. olive oil

1 jalapeño pepper, ribs and seeds removed, and finely diced

2 TB. fresh ginger, minced

1 TB. garlic, minced

1 TB. *curry powder*

½ tsp. sea salt

¼ tsp. freshly ground black pepper

¼ tsp. cayenne

2 cups water or low-sodium vegetable broth

1 (15-oz.) can chickpeas, drained and rinsed

1 (10-oz.) pkg. frozen chopped spinach

1 medium zucchini, cut into quarters lengthwise and thinly sliced

1 cup fresh green beans, cut into 2-in. pieces or frozen cut green beans

1 TB. lemon juice or lime juice

1. In a large saucepan, place Yukon gold potatoes, cover with water, and cook over medium heat for 7 minutes. Add cauliflower, and cook for 3 to 5 more minutes or until potatoes are just tender and can be pierced easily with a knife. Drain vegetables in a colander, and set aside.

2. Place a large pot over medium heat. Add yellow onion and olive oil, and sauté, stirring often, for 3 minutes. Add jalapeño pepper, ginger, garlic, curry powder, sea salt, pepper, and cayenne, and sauté, stirring often, for 2 more minutes.

3. Add potato-cauliflower mixture, water, chickpeas, spinach, zucchini, green beans, and lemon juice, and stir well to combine. Increase heat to high, and bring to a boil. Cover, reduce heat to low, and simmer for 10 to 15 minutes or until vegetables are tender. Remove from heat.

4. Taste and adjust seasonings as desired. Serve over basmati rice or other grains, along with a little vegan yogurt on the side if you need something cool and creamy to offset the heat.

Variation: If you like your curries really hot and spicy, you can add additional curry powder and jalapeño pepper as desired. You also can replace the frozen chopped spinach with 3 cups chopped fresh greens such as kale, Swiss chard, or collard greens.

Plant-Based Dietitian Recommends: Substitute 2 tablespoons coconut water, vegetable broth, or water for the olive oil.

> **DEFINITION**
>
> **Curry powder,** which gets its yellow color from turmeric, is a blend of several spices, including coriander, cinnamon, cumin, cayenne, cardamom, fenugreek, mustard seed, nutmeg, clove, allspice, bay leaf, and black or white pepper. It also may or may not contain salt. You can find mild or hot (also known as madras) curry powders in most grocery and natural foods stores and gourmet specialty markets.

White Pizza with Pesto and Veggies

We've topped this freshly prepared pizza crust with Béchamel Sauce swirled with flavorful pesto, an assortment of arugula, colorful and crisp veggies, black olives, and a generous scattering of Mellow Jack Cheese.

Yield:	Prep time:	Cook time:	Serving size:
1 (12-inch) thick crust, 1 (14-inch) thin crust, or 1 (9×13-inch) rectangular crust or 8 or 9 pieces	15 minutes, plus 1 hour rise time	15 to 20 minutes	1 piece

1 batch Pizza Crust dough (recipe in Chapter 5)

1 cup hot Béchamel Sauce (recipe in Chapter 9)

1 TB. Spicy Sprinkles (recipe in Chapter 6) or nutritional yeast flakes

3 TB. Basil, Spinach, and Pumpkin Seed Pesto (recipe in Chapter 9)

2 cups baby arugula or baby spinach, roughly chopped

$\frac{1}{2}$ cup red onion, cut into 1-in. strips

$\frac{1}{2}$ cup green bell pepper, cut into 1-in. strips

$\frac{1}{2}$ cup red bell pepper, cut into 1-in. strips

$\frac{1}{2}$ cup crimini mushrooms, cut in half and thinly sliced

$\frac{1}{2}$ cup artichoke hearts, roughly chopped

$\frac{1}{4}$ cup kalamata olives or other olives, pitted and roughly chopped

1 cup shredded Mellow Jack Cheese (recipe in Chapter 6)

$\frac{1}{2}$ tsp. dried basil

$\frac{1}{2}$ tsp. crushed red pepper flakes

$\frac{1}{4}$ tsp. freshly ground black pepper

1. Form Pizza Crust dough into desired shape on a baking pan, cover, and set aside to rise in a warm place for 1 hour.

2. Preheat the oven to 450°F.

3. In a small bowl, combine hot Béchamel Sauce and Spicy Sprinkles. Evenly spread Béchamel Sauce mixture over risen pizza crust. Drop spoonfuls of Basil, Spinach, and Pumpkin Seed Pesto over sauce and swirl into a haphazard marbleized pattern.

4. Layer over sauce, in order, arugula, red onion, green bell pepper, red bell pepper, crimini mushrooms, artichoke hearts, and kalamata olives. Scatter shredded Mellow Jack Cheese over vegetables, and sprinkle basil, crushed red pepper flakes, and pepper over top.

5. Bake for 15 to 20 minutes or until pizza crust is crisp and golden brown on the bottom and around the edges and cheese is melted. Remove from the oven. Let cool for several minutes, cut into pieces as desired, and serve hot.

Variation: For a more traditional pizza, replace the Béchamel Sauce with Five-Minute Marinara (recipe in Chapter 9), and top with your favorite vegetables. To make a **Veggie Calzone** (a savory, crescent-shape turnover), after preparing the pizza crust, instead of forming it into the desired shape directly on the baking pan, shape it into a 12- or 14-inch circle on a piece of parchment paper (or use a Silpat liner). Then cover, and let it rise for 1 hour. Assemble all the pizza components and toppings on half of the risen pizza crust, leaving a 2-inch border. With the help of the parchment paper, lift the empty half of the pizza crust up and over to enclose the toppings, press around the edges with a fork to seal, and bake as directed.

CORNUCOPIA

In the United States, *white pizza* refers to a pizza made without tomato sauce. Instead, it's topped with a white sauce, ricotta cheese, or pesto, followed by toppings and cheese. In Italy, pizza made without tomato sauce is called *pizza bianca* and typically consists of a pizza crust topped with olive oil, salt, and some fresh herbs like rosemary or basil.

Mushroom and Marinara Stacks

You could call this a personal mushroom pizza because whole balsamic vinegar–marinated portobello mushroom caps are used much like a pizza crust in this marinara and cheese layered dish.

Yield:	Prep time:	Cook time:	Serving size:
4 mushroom stacks	5 to 7 minutes, plus 10 minutes marinate time	20 to 25 minutes	1 mushroom stack

4 tsp. balsamic vinegar

¼ tsp. garlic powder or garlic granules

4 large portobello mushrooms, stems removed

¾ cup Five-Minute Marinara (recipe in Chapter 9)

1 cup shredded Mellow Jack Cheese or Better Cheddar (recipes in Chapter 6)

4 tsp. Italian Herb Sprinkles (variation in Chapter 6) or Spicy Sprinkles (recipe in Chapter 6) or nutritional yeast flakes

2 TB. fresh basil, cut chiffonade, or 1 tsp. dried basil

1. Preheat the oven to 425°F. Line a cookie sheet with parchment paper or a Silpat liner.

2. In a small bowl, combine balsamic vinegar and garlic powder. Using your fingers, rub ½ teaspoon balsamic vinegar mixture on both top and bottom of each portobello mushroom cap, and place mushroom caps gill side up on the prepared cookie sheet. Set aside for 10 minutes to marinate.

3. Flip over mushroom caps, and bake gill side down for 10 minutes. Remove from the oven. Flip over mushroom caps with a spatula so they're gill side up.

4. Top each mushroom cap with, in order, 3 tablespoons Five-Minute Marinara, ¼ cup shredded Mellow Jack Cheese, 1 teaspoon Italian Herb Sprinkles, and ½ tablespoon basil. Repeat assembly procedure for remaining mushroom caps and filling ingredients.

5. Return portobello mushrooms to the oven, and bake for 10 to 15 more minutes or until mushrooms are tender and cheese is melted. Remove from the oven, and serve hot.

Variation: You can also add other toppings to your mushroom stacks, such as 1 or 2 tablespoons diced red onion or bell peppers, ¼ cup roughly chopped spinach, or a few slices of Savory Sausages (recipe in Chapter 12) for each mushroom.

MEATLESS AND WHEATLESS

This dish makes a tasty option for those concerned with counting carbs. However, you can turn it into a filling sandwich by placing a hot mushroom and marinara stack between 2 slices Multi-Grain Sandwich Bread or a split Gluten-Free Hamburger Bun (recipes in Chapter 5). And for an even more flavorful sandwich, prior to assembling, spread 1 tablespoon Basil, Spinach, and Pumpkin Seed Pesto (recipe in Chapter 9) on each slice of bread or bun.

Black Bean, Sweet Potato, and Sausage Tostadas

These tostadas are made with our Spicy Cilantro-Lime Black Bean Spread; a seasoned mixture of sweet potato, onions, and Savory Sausage; and some of our favorite toppings.

Yield:	Prep time:	Cook time:	Serving size:
12 tostadas	15 to 20 minutes	10 to 15 minutes	1 tostada

1½ cups sweet potatoes, cut into ¼-in. cubes

⅔ cup water

½ cup yellow onion, finely diced

1 TB. garlic, minced

1 Savory Sausage (recipe in Chapter 12), cut into quarters lengthwise and thinly sliced

1 TB. Spicy Sprinkles (recipe in Chapter 6) or nutritional yeast flakes

¾ tsp. chili powder

¼ tsp. ground cumin

¼ tsp. smoked paprika

¼ tsp. freshly ground black pepper

12 corn tostada shells

1½ cups Spicy Cilantro-Lime Black Bean Spread (recipe in Chapter 8)

¾ cup shredded Better Cheddar or Mellow Jack Cheese (recipes in Chapter 6)

2¼ cups loose-leaf lettuce or other lettuce, finely shredded

¾ cup Sausalito Salsa (recipe in Chapter 8) or store-bought salsa

¾ cup Whoo-Pea Guacamole (recipe in Chapter 8) or 1 medium Hass avocado, peeled, pitted, and finely diced

¼ cup Tofu Sour Cream (recipe in Chapter 9) (optional)

1. In a small saucepan, combine sweet potatoes, water, yellow onion, and garlic, and bring to a boil over high heat. Cover, reduce heat to low, and simmer for 5 minutes.

2. Stir in Savory Sausage, Spicy Sprinkles, chili powder, cumin, smoked paprika, and pepper. Cover and cook for 3 to 5 more minutes or until sweet potatoes are tender and most of liquid is absorbed. Remove from heat.

3. While sweet potato mixture is cooking, bake tostada shells according to the package instructions. Remove from the oven.

4. In a small saucepan over medium heat, heat Spicy Cilantro-Lime Black Bean Spread, stirring often, for 2 minutes or until heated through. Alternatively, place spread in a microwave-safe bowl and microwave for 1 or 2 minutes as needed.

5. Spread 2 tablespoons Spicy Cilantro-Lime Black Bean Spread over top of 1 warm tostada shell, and top with 2½ tablespoons sweet potato mixture. Layer over top, in order, 1 tablespoon shredded Better Cheddar, 3 tablespoons shredded lettuce, 1 tablespoon Sausalito Salsa, 1 tablespoon Whoo-Pea Guacamole, and 1 teaspoon Tofu Sour Cream (if using). Repeat assembly procedure for remaining tostada shells and other components. Serve hot.

Variation: For an easier preparation, replace the Spicy Cilantro-Lime Black Bean Spread with 1 (16-ounce) can vegetarian refried beans.

MEATLESS AND WHEATLESS

This recipe can be adapted easily to many different interpretations. If you're in the mood for some crunchy tacos instead, replace the baked tostada shells with baked yellow corn or blue corn taco shells. Or for soft tacos, instead use warm brown rice, hemp, or other gluten-free tortillas. If you want to take it on the go, simply roll up all the ingredients in the tortillas burrito-style.

Shepherdess' Pie

This meatless version of the classic comfort food has a bottom layer made with vegetables, mushrooms, and tempeh in a red wine and tomato gravy, all covered in a blanket of mashed potatoes.

Yield:	Prep time:	Cook time:	Serving size:
1 (9×13-inch) pan or 12 cups	40 to 45 minutes	35 to 40 minutes	1½ cups

2 lb. (about 6 cups) Yukon gold potatoes, peeled and cut into 2-in. pieces

⅓ cup soy milk or other nondairy milk

1 TB. nonhydrogenated margarine

1½ tsp. sea salt

1 tsp. freshly ground black pepper

2 cups turnips or parsnips, peeled and cut into 1-in. pieces

1 cup celery, thinly sliced

1 cup yellow onion, diced

1½ TB. olive oil

1 (8-oz.) pkg. tempeh

1½ cups crimini mushrooms or other mushrooms, cut in half and thinly sliced

2 TB. garlic, minced

1 (10-oz.) pkg. frozen mixed vegetables blend (carrots, corn, green beans, and peas)

1½ tsp. dried basil

1½ tsp. dried thyme

1 tsp. rubbed sage

3 cups low-sodium vegetable broth

⅓ cup red wine

2 TB. tomato paste

1½ TB. wheat-free tamari

1½ TB. gluten-free flour of choice

⅓ cup chopped fresh parsley

1. Place Yukon gold potatoes in a large saucepan, cover with water, and cook over medium heat for 15 to 20 minutes or until potatoes are tender. Remove from heat. Reserve ⅓ cup cooking liquid, drain potatoes in a colander, and return potatoes to the saucepan.

2. To potatoes, add soy milk, reserved cooking liquid, margarine, ½ teaspoon sea salt, and ¼ teaspoon pepper. Using a potato masher, mash potato mixture until smooth, and set aside.

3. Preheat the oven to 425°F.

4. Meanwhile, place a large, nonstick skillet over medium heat. Add turnips, celery, yellow onion, and olive oil, and sauté, stirring often, for 7 minutes.

5. Using your fingers, crumble tempeh into the skillet. Add crimini mushrooms and garlic, and sauté, stirring often, for 5 more minutes.

6. Add frozen mixed vegetables, basil, thyme, rubbed sage, remaining 1 teaspoon sea salt, and remaining ¾ teaspoon pepper, and sauté, stirring often, for 3 more minutes or until turnips are tender.

7. In a medium bowl, whisk together vegetable broth, red wine, tomato paste, tamari, and flour. Stir mixture into the skillet, and cook for 1 or 2 minutes or until thickened. Stir in parsley. Remove from heat. Transfer skillet mixture to a 9×13-inch baking pan or large casserole dish.

8. Drop spoonfuls of mashed potatoes over filling mixture and gently spread to completely cover top and seal edges of casserole. Using a fork, rake surface of mashed potatoes.

9. Bake for 15 to 20 minutes or until filling is bubbling hot and mashed potatoes are dry and a little browned. Remove from the oven, and serve hot.

Variation: For a more flavorful topping, replace the mashed potatoes mixture with Mmm Mmm Mashed Potatoes (recipe in Chapter 18).

Plant-Based Dietitian Recommends: Use unsweetened plant-based milk. Substitute an extra 2 tablespoons reserved liquid, soy milk, or vegetable broth for the margarine. Or use ¼ cup vegetable broth or water for the olive oil in the sauté.

MEATLESS AND WHEATLESS

Typically a meat-based shepherd's pie is made with mutton, lamb, or beef. If you're not in the mood for tempeh, replace it with 2 cups chopped Beef-Style Gluten-Free Seitan (variation in Chapter 12). To give the gravy a richer flavor, add an additional 1 tablespoon wheat-free tamari. And why *Shepherdess'* Pie? Because this recipe was developed by women!

Seitan Divan

Our veganized divan casserole features chunks of our gluten-free seitan, broccoli, and an enhanced Béchamel Sauce, all topped with breadcrumbs.

Yield:	Prep time:	Cook time:	Serving size:
6 cups	10 to 15 minutes	25 to 30 minutes	1½ cups

2 cups hot Béchamel Sauce (recipe in Chapter 9)

2 TB. white wine

2 TB. nutritional yeast flakes

1 TB. Dijon mustard

1 slice Multi-Grain Sandwich Bread (recipe in Chapter 5)

1 lb. frozen broccoli florets or 1 medium bunch broccoli, cut into small florets or 3-in. spears

2 cups Chicken-Style Gluten-Free Seitan (recipe in Chapter 12), cut into bite-size chunks

½ cup shredded Better Cheddar (recipe in Chapter 6)

Smoked paprika or sweet paprika

1. In a large bowl, combine hot Béchamel Sauce, white wine, nutritional yeast flakes, and Dijon mustard, and stir well. Set aside.

2. Preheat the oven to 375°F. Lightly oil a 9×13-inch baking pan or large casserole dish, or use a silicone baking pan.

3. In a food processor fitted with an S blade, place slice of Multi-Grain Sandwich Bread, and process for 1 minute or until you get fine crumbs. Measure out ½ cup breadcrumbs (save any extra for use in another recipe), and set aside.

4. Place broccoli in bottom of the prepared baking dish. Place Chicken-Style Gluten-Free Seitan chunks on top of broccoli, and pour Béchamel Sauce mixture over top. Evenly sprinkle Better Cheddar over sauce, and top with reserved breadcrumbs. Finish with a light sprinkling of smoked paprika over top.

5. Bake for 20 to 25 minutes or until sauce is bubbling hot. Remove from the oven, and serve hot, with individual servings over cooked brown rice or other grains as desired.

Variation: You can replace the Chicken-Style Gluten-Free Seitan with 8 ounces tofu or tempeh, cut into 1-inch strips, and the Béchamel Sauce with Roasted Onion and Garlic Gravy (recipe in Chapter 9).

CORNUCOPIA

Seitan (pronounced *say-tahn*)—also referred to as wheat-meat, wheat gluten, or simply gluten—was developed by Buddhist monks as a meat substitute. It's known for having a chewy, meatlike texture and flavor when cooked properly and well seasoned. Our gluten-free version is very similar in texture to its wheat-based counterpart—so much so, in fact, that we suggest you try it as a replacement in other gluten-free vegan recipes that call for seitan.

Gratifying Grains

In This Chapter

- International rice dishes
- Marvelous millet mixtures
- Colorful quinoa concoctions

For centuries, grains have been the staple of the daily diet for countless cultures throughout the world. Humankind has survived and thrived by centering their diet on rice, quinoa, barley, millet, teff, and other whole grains. The term *whole* grain basically means that the bran, germ, and endosperm of the complete grain kernel are still intact and haven't been removed or polished away. When eaten in this form, your body can utilize the wealth of nutrients offered in these tiny powerhouses, including fiber, starch, protein, iron, selenium, manganese, magnesium, as well as many beneficial B vitamins, such as folate, thiamine, niacin, riboflavin, and pantothenic acid.

If you just boil your grains in water, they can taste a bit blah, but you can easily and quickly remedy this by replacing the water with vegetable broth, fruit juices, or other flavorful liquids. Feel free to liberally season them with herbs, spices, nutritional yeast flakes, sea salt, and black pepper and to combine them with cooked beans; fresh, frozen, or canned vegetables; and nuts and seeds to your heart's content.

The most affordable way to purchase your whole grains is from bulk bins in your local health food store. If you don't go through them quickly, store them in airtight containers to avoid attracting bugs.

Aloha Pineapple Rice

This cheerfully colorful rice dish, sweetened by pineapples with a macadamia nut crunch, is a luau in a bowl. With one bite, you'll feel like you suddenly landed on the beautiful beaches of Hawaii.

Yield:	Prep time:	Cook time:	Serving size:
8 cups	15 to 20 minutes	15 to 20 minutes	1½ cups

¾ cup Date Paste (recipe in Chapter 8)

⅓ cup wheat-free tamari

⅓ cup brown rice vinegar

2 TB. fresh ginger, minced

2 large garlic cloves, minced

1 tsp. crushed red pepper flakes

½ cup unsweetened coconut water

1 medium white onion, diced

1 cup carrots, diced

1 cup celery, diced

1 cup red bell pepper, diced

4 cups cooked brown rice

½ cup soy milk

2 cups pineapple tidbits

¾ cup raw macadamia nuts, roughly chopped

1. In a blender, place Date Paste, tamari, brown rice vinegar, ginger, garlic, and crushed red pepper flakes, and blend for 1 minute. Scrape down the sides of the container with a spatula, and blend for 15 more seconds.

2. In a large pot over medium-high heat, combine coconut water and white onion, and sauté, stirring often, for 3 to 5 minutes or until onion is soft.

3. Add carrots, celery, and red bell pepper, and sauté, stirring often, for 2 more minutes.

4. Add brown rice, soy milk, Date Paste mixture, pineapple tidbits, and macadamia nuts, and bring to a boil over high heat. Reduce heat to low, and simmer for 5 minutes. Remove from heat, and serve hot or at room temperature as desired.

Variation: Turn this dish into fast food by using a commercial wheat-free teriyaki sauce. Instead of making the sauce in the blender, substitute ¾ cup store-bought teriyaki sauce and use in place of step 1.

CORNUCOPIA

For quick rice dishes, try precooked brown rice packets in the freezer sections of your local grocery and natural foods stores. Pop them in the microwave, and in 3 minutes, you've got ready-to-eat brown rice!

Black Forbidden Rice with Mango, Bell Peppers, and Cashews

This strikingly beautiful and tasty Asian-inspired rice dish features *black forbidden rice*, sweet and juicy pieces of mango, red and orange bell peppers, crunchy cashews, and cilantro.

Yield:	Prep time:	Cook time:	Serving size:
5 to 6 cups	10 to 15 minutes	30 minutes	1 cup

1¾ cups water

1 cup black forbidden rice

¾ tsp. sea salt

½ tsp. freshly ground black pepper or garlic pepper

½ cup raw cashews

1 large mango, peeled, pitted, and cut into ½-in. cubes

¾ cup red bell pepper, cut into ½-in. cubes

¾ cup orange or yellow bell pepper, cut into ½-in. cubes

⅓ cup green onion, thinly sliced

⅓ cup chopped fresh cilantro

1 TB. wheat-free tamari

1½ tsp. toasted sesame oil

½ tsp. crushed red pepper flakes

1. In a medium saucepan, combine water, black forbidden rice, sea salt, and pepper, and bring to a boil over high heat. Cover, reduce heat to low, and simmer for 30 minutes or until water is absorbed. Remove from heat and set aside for 5 minutes to steam.

2. Preheat the oven to 350°F.

3. Place cashews in a pie pan or baking pan. Bake for 5 to 10 minutes or until cashews are golden brown. Remove from the oven and set aside.

4. Fluff black forbidden rice with a fork to loosen grains. Add mango, red bell pepper, orange bell pepper, green onion, cilantro, toasted cashews, tamari, toasted sesame oil, and crushed red pepper flakes, and stir well to combine. Serve hot or at room temperature as desired.

Variation: To turn this side dish into a one-plate meal, serve individual portions on top of baby spinach or mixed baby greens. If you can't find black forbidden rice, you can use wild rice instead, but increase water to 3 cups and simmer for 40 to 45 minutes or until wild rice is just tender.

> **DEFINITION**
>
> **Black forbidden rice** is a short-grain heirloom rice variety that has a deep, purplish-black color with a slightly nutty flavor. According to legend, this stunning and fragrant rice was cultivated exclusively for the emperors of China to enrich their health and ensure their longevity, hence the name black forbidden rice. Find it packaged or in bulk bins in grocery and natural foods stores.

Vegetable Biryani

You don't need to go to your local Indian restaurant when you're in the mood for spicy vegetable biryani. With a visit to your local grocery or natural foods store, you can find all the spices you need for this fragrant and flavorful dish.

Yield:	Prep time:	Cook time:	Serving size:
4 cups	8 to 10 minutes	30 to 40 minutes	1 cup

⅔ cup yellow onion, diced

1 small red chile or green chile pepper, ribs and seeds removed, and finely diced

1 TB. garlic, minced

1 TB. fresh ginger, minced

2 tsp. olive oil or other oil

1 tsp. curry powder

½ tsp. cardamom seeds

½ tsp. mustard seeds

½ tsp. ground cinnamon

½ tsp. ground coriander

½ tsp. ground cumin

½ tsp. sea salt

¼ tsp. freshly ground black pepper

2 cups water

1 cup basmati rice

⅔ cup red bell pepper, diced

⅔ cup frozen peas

⅓ cup raisins

1. In a medium saucepan, combine yellow onion, red chile, garlic, ginger, and olive oil, and sauté over medium heat, stirring often, for 3 minutes.

2. Add curry powder, cardamom seeds, mustard seeds, cinnamon, coriander, cumin, sea salt, and pepper, and sauté, stirring often, for 2 or 3 more minutes or until spices are fragrant.

3. Stir in water and basmati rice, increase heat to high, and bring to a boil. Cover, reduce heat to low, and simmer for 25 to 35 minutes or until all liquid is absorbed. Remove from heat and set aside for 5 minutes to steam.

4. Fluff basmati rice with a fork to loosen grains. Add red bell pepper, peas, and raisins, and stir well to combine. Taste and adjust seasonings as desired. Serve hot.

Variation: For an even more veggie-studded biryani, replace the red bell pepper with ¾ cup cauliflower florets and the frozen peas with ¾ cup frozen mixed vegetable blend (carrots, corn, peas, and green beans), but add this alternate combination of vegetables to rice mixture prior to simmering.

Plant-Based Dietitian Recommends: Substitute 2 tablespoons coconut water, vegetable broth, or water for the oil.

CORNUCOPIA

Cardamom is available in three forms: ground powder, cardamom seeds, and whole cardamom pods. If you can only find whole cardamom pods, to access the cardamom seeds contained inside, place cardamom pods on a cutting board, firmly crush them with the bottom of a skillet until the pods crack open, and peel away the outer pods with your fingers to expose the seeds.

Winter Squash Risotto

The flavors of sweet winter squash and savory sage play well off each other as well as the creamy and chewy *arborio rice*, and our Spicy Sprinkles add a bit of cheesiness to this Italian-style risotto.

Yield:	Prep time:	Cook time:	Serving size:
5 or 6 cups	8 to 10 minutes	25 to 30 minutes	1 cup as a side dish or 1½ cups as a main dish

2 cups low-sodium vegetable broth

1½ cups water

4 cups winter squash (such as acorn, butternut, buttercup, kabocha, etc.), peeled, seeds removed, and cut into ½-in. cubes

¾ cup shallots or yellow onion, finely diced

2 TB. garlic, minced

2 tsp. olive oil

1 cup arborio rice

2 TB. chopped fresh sage or ½ tsp. rubbed sage

½ tsp. sea salt

¼ tsp. freshly ground black pepper or garlic pepper

⅓ cup white wine

1 TB. Bragg Liquid Aminos or wheat-free tamari

¼ cup Spicy Sprinkles (recipe in Chapter 6) or Italian Herb Sprinkles (variation in Chapter 6) or nutritional yeast flakes

¼ cup chopped fresh parsley (preferably Italian flat-leaf parsley)

1. In a small saucepan, combine vegetable broth and water, cover, and bring to a simmer over low heat.

2. In a large saucepan, combine winter squash, shallots, garlic, and olive oil, and sauté over medium heat, stirring often, for 3 minutes. Add arborio rice, sage, sea salt, and pepper, and sauté, stirring often, for 2 or 3 more minutes or until sage is fragrant.

3. Add white wine and Bragg Liquid Aminos, and cook, stirring often, until wine is almost completely absorbed. Add 1 cup vegetable stock mixture, and cook, stirring often, until completely absorbed. Continue stirring and adding vegetable broth mixture 1 cup at a time, allowing each addition to be fully absorbed before adding the next, for 15 to 20 minutes or until arborio rice is tender and creamy-looking but still slightly firm.

4. Reduce heat to low. Add Spicy Sprinkles and parsley, and continue to cook, stirring often, for 3 to 5 more minutes or until very creamy but not runny. Remove from heat. Taste and adjust seasonings as desired. Top individual servings with additional Spicy Sprinkles as desired, and serve.

Variation: You can replace the winter squash with an equal amount of diced sweet potatoes or garnet yams and the fresh sage with ¼ cup fresh basil, chopped or cut chiffonade. If you can't find arborio rice, you can use short-grain brown rice.

Plant-Based Dietitian Recommends: Substitute 2 tablespoons vegetable broth or water for the oil.

> **DEFINITION**
>
> **Arborio rice** is a plump, Italian variety of short-grain rice. The individual grains of arborio rice have a lot of starch in their outer layers that dissolves when cooked in a large amount of liquid, resulting in a thick and creamy sauce, yet the center of the rice retains its firm and chewy texture. These creamy-chewy characteristics make it the best choice for preparing a risotto.

Golden Cauliflower and Millet Mash

Trying to get your kids to eat more vegetables? By cooking and mashing together wholesome *millet* with orange cauliflower, you can pull a fast one on them, making them think this is mashed potatoes.

Yield:	Prep time:	Cook time:	Serving size:
5 or 6 cups	5 to 7 minutes	30 to 35 minutes	1 cup

1½ cups millet

1 cup yellow onion or shallots, diced

2 cups low-sodium vegetable broth

1 medium head orange cauliflower, cut into small florets

2 cups water

1 tsp. sea salt

½ tsp. garlic powder or garlic granules

½ tsp. white pepper, garlic pepper, or freshly ground black pepper

2 TB. nutritional yeast flakes

1. Place a large saucepan over medium heat. Add millet, and cook, stirring often, for 2 or 3 minutes or until it begins to "pop" and some grains appear lightly browned. Transfer toasted millet to a small bowl, and set aside.

2. Return the saucepan to medium heat. Add yellow onion and ½ cup vegetable broth, and sauté, stirring often, for 3 minutes.

3. Add cauliflower, water, toasted millet, remaining 1½ cups vegetable broth, sea salt, garlic powder, and white pepper. Increase heat to high, and bring to a boil. Cover, reduce heat to low, and simmer for 25 to 30 minutes or until cauliflower and millet are tender and liquid is absorbed. Remove from heat.

4. Using a potato masher, mash millet mixture until as smooth or chunky as desired. If needed, add a little additional water to achieve desired consistency. Alternatively, beat millet mixture with an electric mixer.

5. Stir in nutritional yeast flakes. Taste and adjust seasonings as desired, and serve hot.

Variation: This mash is tasty served plain or topped with Roasted Onion and Garlic Gravy (recipe in Chapter 9). If you can't find orange cauliflower, use fresh white cauliflower or 1 (16-ounce) package frozen cauliflower florets.

Mean, Green Millet

This spicy, green grain side dish is the perfect accompaniment to any Mexican-style meal, and it's a great way to sneak spinach past finicky eaters who claim they can't stand it.

Yield:	Prep time:	Cook time:	Serving size:
4 cups	10 to 15 minutes	40 to 45 minutes	1 cup

1 cup millet

½ cup yellow onion or shallots, finely diced

1¾ cups low-sodium vegetable broth

1½ TB. garlic, minced

1 cup soy milk or other nondairy milk

1 cup baby spinach, tightly packed

½ cup fresh cilantro leaves, tightly packed

2 jalapeño peppers or serrano chile peppers, ribs and seeds removed, and diced

1 TB. nutritional yeast flakes

1 tsp. sea salt

½ tsp. freshly ground black pepper or garlic pepper

½ cup frozen peas

⅓ cup green onion, thinly sliced

1. Place a large saucepan over medium heat. Add millet and cook, stirring often, for 2 or 3 minutes or until it begins to "pop" and some grains appear lightly browned. Transfer toasted millet to a small bowl, and set aside.

2. Return the saucepan to medium heat. Add yellow onion, ¼ cup vegetable broth, and garlic, and sauté, stirring often, for 3 minutes.

3. Meanwhile, in a blender, combine soy milk, remaining 1½ cups vegetable broth, spinach, cilantro, jalapeño peppers, nutritional yeast flakes, sea salt, and pepper, and blend for 1 or 2 minutes or until smooth. Scrape down the sides of the container with a spatula, and blend for 15 more seconds.

4. Add soy milk mixture and toasted millet to the saucepan, and bring to a boil over high heat. Cover, reduce heat to low, and simmer for 30 to 35 minutes or until all liquid is absorbed. Remove from heat.

5. Fluff millet mixture with a fork to loosen grains. Add peas and green onion, and stir well to combine. Taste and adjust seasonings as desired. Serve hot.

Variation: For **Arroz Verde,** replace the millet with basmati rice, but skip the toasting step. After the rice has been fluffed, add an additional $\frac{1}{4}$ cup chopped fresh cilantro and 1 cup finely chopped spinach.

AGAINST THE GRAIN

When working with jalapeño peppers or other hot chile peppers, avoid touching your eyes or face; otherwise, you'll experience tremendous burning at the point of contact, and your eyes may begin to water profusely. Don a pair of disposable vinyl gloves (food handler's gloves) for added safety from the fiery hot inner ribs and seeds.

Mixed Grain Pilaf

This savory pilaf is prepared with earthy crimini mushrooms, celery, shallots, and a blend of several different varieties of rice, buckwheat groats, and quinoa.

Yield:	Prep time:	Cook time:	Serving size:
5 cups	10 to 15 minutes	50 to 55 minutes	1 cup

1/3 cup quinoa or millet

2/3 cup plus 1 1/2 cups water

1 1/3 cups crimini mushrooms or other mushrooms, cut in half and thinly sliced

2/3 cup celery, diced

2/3 cup shallots or yellow onion, diced

2 TB. garlic, minced

1 1/2 tsp. olive oil or other oil

1 cup mixed rice and wild rice blend

1/3 cup toasted buckwheat groats (or kasha)

1 1/2 tsp. dried thyme

1 tsp. rubbed sage

1 tsp. sea salt

1/2 tsp. freshly ground black pepper or garlic pepper

2 cups low-sodium vegetable broth

1 bay leaf

1/3 cup green onion, thinly sliced

1/3 cup chopped fresh parsley (preferably Italian flat-leaf parsley)

2 tsp. Bragg Liquid Aminos or wheat-free tamari

1. Place quinoa in a fine mesh sieve, and rinse well under running water for 1 minute. Place 2/3 cup water and quinoa in a small saucepan, and bring to a boil over high heat. Cover, reduce heat to low, and simmer for 18 to 20 minutes or until quinoa is tender and all liquid is absorbed. Remove from heat and set aside.

2. Meanwhile, in a large saucepan over medium heat, combine crimini mushrooms, celery, shallots, garlic, and olive oil, and sauté, stirring often, for 3 minutes. Add mixed rice and wild rice blend, buckwheat groats, thyme, sage, sea salt, and pepper, and sauté, stirring often, for 2 minutes.

3. Add vegetable broth, remaining 1 1/2 cups water, and bay leaf, and bring to a boil over high heat. Cover, reduce heat to low, and simmer for 40 to 45 minutes or until grains are tender and all liquid is absorbed. Remove from heat, and remove and discard bay leaf.

4. Fluff mixed rice mixture and quinoa with a fork to loosen grains. Add quinoa to rice mixture along with green onion, parsley, and Bragg Liquid Aminos, and stir gently to combine. Serve hot.

Variation: For a splash of color and texture, add 2 cups chopped spinach or lacinato kale and ¹/₂ cup toasted sliced almonds.

> **MEATLESS AND WHEATLESS**
>
> When making a pilaf, the rice is sautéed in oil to help keep the grains fluffy and separated during the final cooking process. And using a mixed rice blend rather than just brown rice is an easy and great-tasting way to get more grains into your daily diet. For making this pilaf, we suggest using Lundberg Wild Blend, which contains long-grain brown, sweet brown, Wehani, Black Japonica, and wild rice varieties.

Ruby Quinoa

This stunning side dish utilizes fresh beet greens (which might be a new ingredient for you) briefly sautéed with red onion, garlic, and herbs and combined with cooked quinoa to tint it a beautiful ruby red color.

Yield:	Prep time:	Cook time:	Serving size:
4 or 5 cups	10 to 15 minutes	20 to 25 minutes	1 cup

1¹/₂ cups quinoa	1 tsp. dried basil
3 cups water	1 tsp. dried thyme
1 large bunch beets, greens still attached	1 TB. nutritional yeast flakes
²/₃ cup red or yellow onion, diced	³/₄ tsp. sea salt
¹/₃ cup low-sodium vegetable broth	¹/₂ tsp. freshly ground black pepper
1¹/₂ TB. garlic, minced	¹/₂ tsp. crushed red pepper flakes (optional)

1. Place quinoa in a fine mesh sieve and rinse well under running water for 1 minute. Place water and quinoa in a medium saucepan, and bring to a boil over high heat. Cover, reduce heat to low, and simmer for 18 to 20 minutes or until quinoa is tender and all liquid is absorbed. Remove from heat.

2. While quinoa is cooking, separate beets and beet greens by cutting greens about 1 inch above beets. Place whole beets in a bag, and store in the refrigerator for use in another recipe. Cut beet greens lengthwise to separate leaves and stems, wash each thoroughly, and place in a colander to drain. Cut stems into 1-inch pieces, roughly chop beet leaves, and place both side by side on a large plate.

3. Place a large, nonstick skillet over medium heat. Add red onion and vegetable broth, and sauté, stirring often, for 2 minutes. Add beet stems, and sauté, stirring often, for 2 more minutes. Add garlic, basil, and thyme, and sauté, stirring often, for 1 more minute.

4. Add beet leaves, nutritional yeast flakes, sea salt, pepper, and crushed red pepper flakes (if using), and sauté, stirring often, for 1 or 2 minutes or until vegetables are tender. Remove from heat.

5. Fluff quinoa with a fork to loosen grains. Add quinoa to the skillet, and stir gently to combine. Taste and adjust seasonings as desired, and serve hot.

Variation: For extra flavor and texture, add $\frac{1}{4}$ cup toasted pine nuts and 1 cup canned chickpeas. If you can't find beets with the greens still attached, substitute $\frac{1}{2}$ cup shredded beets, and either 4 large leaves rainbow Swiss chard or lacinato kale, roughly chopped.

CORNUCOPIA

When you buy fresh beets by the bunch, with the greens still attached, you're actually getting two items for the price of one. Thinly slice the beet stems; dice, slice, or shred the beets; and use them either raw or cooked in recipes as desired. Beet greens are quite tasty and incredibly nutritious. Small and tender beet leaves can be left whole and eaten raw in salads, while more mature or tough leaves are best cut crosswise into thin strips for use in soups, stews, side dishes, casseroles, and even stir-fries.

Spanish-Style Quinoa

When you're in the mood for some Spanish rice, don't just open up a boxed mix! Change things up a bit, and make it from scratch with this spicy quinoa-based recipe instead!

Yield:	Prep time:	Cook time:	Serving size:
4 or 5 servings	10 to 15 minutes	30 to 35 minutes	1 cup

½ cup yellow onion, diced

½ cup green bell pepper, diced

¾ cup low-sodium vegetable broth or water

1 TB. garlic, minced

1 cup quinoa

1 (14-oz.) can fire-roasted petite-cut diced tomatoes with chipotle peppers

1 tsp. chili powder

1 tsp. dried oregano

½ tsp. ground cumin

½ tsp. smoked paprika or sweet paprika

½ tsp. sea salt

¼ tsp. freshly ground black pepper or garlic pepper

¼ cup green onion, thinly sliced

¼ cup chopped fresh cilantro or parsley

1. Place a medium saucepan over medium heat. Add yellow onion, green bell pepper, and ¼ cup vegetable broth, and sauté, stirring often, for 3 minutes. Add garlic, and sauté, stirring often, for 1 more minute.

2. Place quinoa in a fine mesh sieve and rinse well under running water for 1 minute. Add quinoa, fire-roasted diced tomatoes, remaining ½ cup vegetable broth, chili powder, oregano, cumin, smoked paprika, sea salt, and pepper, and bring to a boil over high heat. Cover, reduce heat to low, and simmer for 22 to 25 minutes or until quinoa is tender and all liquid is absorbed. Stir in green onion and chopped cilantro. Remove from heat.

3. Fluff quinoa with a fork to loosen grains. Taste and adjust seasonings as desired, and serve hot.

Variation: If you can't find petite diced tomatoes, use 1 (14-ounce) can diced tomatoes. For extra flavor, use tomatoes with green chiles added. For a heartier side dish, add 1 cup canned beans of choice.

Red Quinoa-Polenta

Ancient Harvest sells logs of precooked polenta with bits of red quinoa mixed in, and that was the inspiration for this homemade concoction of creamy polenta, red quinoa, and fresh basil.

Yield:	Prep time:	Cook time:	Serving size:
6 cups	3 to 5 minutes	40 to 45 minutes	1 cup

6 cups water

1 cup medium- or coarse-grind yellow cornmeal

$\frac{1}{2}$ cup Inca red quinoa

$1\frac{1}{4}$ tsp. sea salt

$\frac{1}{2}$ tsp. freshly ground black pepper or garlic pepper

$\frac{1}{3}$ cup fresh basil, cut *chiffonade*

$\frac{1}{4}$ cup chopped fresh parsley (preferably Italian flat-leaf parsley)

$1\frac{1}{2}$ TB. Italian Herb Sprinkles (variation in Chapter 6) or Spicy Sprinkles (recipe in Chapter 6), or nutritional yeast flakes

1. In a large pot, place water, and bring to a boil over high heat. Slowly add cornmeal, whisking constantly to prevent lumps. Continue to whisk for 1 or 2 minutes or until mixture begins to boil again. Reduce heat to very low. Cover and simmer for 10 minutes.

2. Place red quinoa in a fine mesh sieve, and rinse well under running water for 1 minute. After water and cornmeal have cooked for 10 minutes, stir in red quinoa, sea salt, and pepper, and continue to cook, stirring every 10 minutes with a long-handled spoon, for 20 to 25 more minutes or until very thick and polenta starts to pull away from the sides of the pot.

3. Add basil, parsley, and Italian Herb Sprinkles, and stir well to combine. Remove from heat, top individual servings with additional Italian Herb Sprinkles as desired, and serve hot.

Variation: If you can find it in your local store, you can replace the red quinoa with black quinoa or a mixed blend of white, red, and black quinoa.

> **DEFINITION**
>
> **Chiffonade** in French means "made from rags." In cooking, chiffonade is a technique for slicing herbs and leafy green vegetables into long, thin, ribbonlike strips. To chiffonade something, stack and roll a small pile of leaves; slice the roll crosswise into fine, thin strips; and gently toss the strips with your fingers to separate them.

Kasha Varnishkas

This classic Jewish dish commonly calls for an egg, but our vegan version tastes delicious without it. If you can't find gluten-free bow-tie pasta, use whatever shape of gluten-free pasta you have on hand.

Yield:	Prep time:	Cook time:	Serving size:
6 cups	5 minutes	25 minutes	1½ cups

1 cup yellow onion, diced

2 cups low-sodium vegetable broth

1½ TB. garlic, minced

1 cup *toasted buckwheat groats* (or kasha)

1½ cups gluten-free bow-tie or other shaped pasta

¼ cup chopped fresh parsley

1 TB. Bragg Liquid Aminos or wheat-free tamari

Sea salt

Freshly ground black pepper

1. In a medium saucepan, combine yellow onion, ¼ cup vegetable broth, and garlic, and cook over medium heat, stirring often, for 3 minutes. Add toasted buckwheat groats, and cook, stirring often, for 1 more minute.

2. Add remaining 1¾ cups vegetable broth, and bring to a boil over high heat. Cover, reduce heat to low, and simmer for 20 minutes or until buckwheat groats are tender and all liquid is absorbed. Remove from heat.

3. Meanwhile, fill a large saucepan $\frac{2}{3}$ full of water, and bring to a boil over medium-high heat. Add bow-ties, and cook, stirring occasionally, according to the package directions or until al dente. Drain bow-ties in a colander, but do not rinse.

4. Fluff buckwheat groats mixture with a fork to loosen grains. Add cooked bow-ties, parsley, and Bragg Liquid Aminos, and stir well to combine. Taste and season with sea salt and pepper as desired, and serve hot.

Variation: You can also add 1 cup sliced crimini mushrooms to the cooking onion mixture, but add an additional $\frac{1}{4}$ cup vegetable broth, too.

DEFINITION

Toasted buckwheat groats (a.k.a. kasha) have been roasted to give them a slightly nutty aroma and flavor. They can be cooked in water or other liquid for eating as a hot cereal or used to make varnishkas, pilafs, knishes, and blintzes. Find them packaged in bulk bins in most grocery and natural foods stores.

Luscious Legumes

In This Chapter

- Spicy legume recipes
- Skillet-sautéed bean dishes
- Slow-cooked bean pots

Lentils, all beans, and peas can be a vegan's nutritional best friend—they really do a body good! Regardless of what form you buy them in—fresh, frozen, canned, or dried—beans and legumes are affordable and offer a tremendous amount of nutritional "bang for your buck." They're excellent sources of fat-free protein, starch, dietary fiber, and numerous vitamins and minerals. Known to prevent cancer, stabilize blood sugar, and keep you full, beans and other legumes are worth their weight in diamonds.

If you're worried you're not amply fulfilling your nutritional needs (or concerned about your family's), you can easily sneak in all your required nutrients via legume-based dishes. By combining them with a few simple ingredients and blending, the humble bean or legume can be transformed into delicious dips and spreads.

In this chapter, you learn how to make Italian- and French-style bean and legume dishes like Cannellini Beans with Escarole and Green Beans Amandine. All-American regional standards and veganized revamps like Mardi Gras Red Beans, Soy-Catash, and everyone's favorite BBQ Baked Beans are also included.

Cannellini Beans with Escarole

You're going to love this classic Italian combination of bitter *escarole* and creamy cannellini beans. It's also tasty served over cooked gluten-free pasta.

Yield:	Prep time:	Cook time:	Serving size:
4 or 5 cups	8 to 10 minutes	1 to 1½ hours	1 cup

6 cups water

1 cup dried cannellini beans, sorted and rinsed

1 bay leaf

1 cup yellow onion, diced

¾ cup low-sodium vegetable broth

2 TB. garlic, minced

1 medium head escarole, torn or cut into bite-size pieces

2 tsp. Italian seasoning blend or ¾ tsp. each dried basil, oregano, and thyme

¾ tsp. sea salt

½ tsp. freshly ground black pepper or garlic pepper

½ tsp. crushed red pepper flakes

¼ cup chopped fresh parsley (preferably Italian flat-leaf parsley)

2 TB. Italian Herb Sprinkles (variation in Chapter 6) or Spicy Sprinkles (recipe in Chapter 6) or nutritional yeast flakes

1. In a large pot, combine water, cannellini beans, and bay leaf, and bring to a boil over high heat. Cover, reduce heat to low, and simmer, stirring occasionally, for 1 to 1½ hours or until cannellini beans are tender. Remove and discard bay leaf.

2. Meanwhile, place a large, nonstick skillet over medium heat. Add yellow onion, ¼ cup vegetable broth, and garlic, and cook, stirring often, for 3 minutes.

3. Add escarole, remaining ½ cup vegetable broth, Italian seasoning blend, sea salt, pepper, and crushed red pepper flakes, and cook, stirring often, for 3 minutes. Cover, reduce heat to low, and simmer for 5 minutes or until escarole is tender. Remove from heat.

4. When cannellini beans are tender, add escarole mixture, parsley, and Italian Herb Sprinkles, and stir well to combine. Remove from heat. Taste and adjust seasonings as desired, top individual servings with additional Italian Herb Sprinkles as desired, and serve hot.

Variation: For a heartier dish, add 1 cup Tempeh Italiano (recipe in Chapter 12). If you can't find dried cannellini beans, you can replace them with Great Northern beans.

DEFINITION

Escarole is a variety of endive, which has very broad, bitter-tasting leaves. It's high in dietary fiber, folic acid, and vitamins A and K, and can be eaten raw in salads, blanched or boiled in water, or sautéed. A medium head of escarole usually yields about 7 cups torn leaves.

Cajun Beans and Greens

Our Savory Sausages elevate the flavor of this spicy, protein-rich dish of canned red beans, collard greens, kale, and aromatic vegetables.

Yield:	Prep time:	Cook time:	Serving size:
4 or 5 cups	15 to 20 minutes	20 to 25 minutes	1 cup

1 cup red or yellow onion, diced

1 cup red bell pepper, diced

1 jalapeño pepper, ribs and seeds removed, and finely diced

1½ cups low-sodium vegetable broth

2 TB. garlic, minced

1 bunch collard greens, stems removed, and roughly chopped

1 bunch green or purple kale, stems removed, and roughly chopped

2 Savory Sausages (recipe in Chapter 12), cut in half lengthwise and thinly sliced

1 (15-oz.) can red beans, pinto beans, or butter beans, drained and rinsed

1 TB. Spicy Sprinkles (recipe in Chapter 6) or nutritional yeast flakes

1 TB. chili powder

1 tsp. dried oregano

1 tsp. dried thyme

½ tsp. sea salt

½ tsp. freshly ground black pepper

¼ tsp. hot pepper sauce or cayenne

1. Place a large pot over medium heat. Add red onion, red bell pepper, jalapeño pepper, ½ cup vegetable broth, and garlic, and cook, stirring often, for 5 minutes.

2. Add remaining 1 cup vegetable broth, and bring to a boil over medium heat. In batches, add collard greens and kale, covering the pot in between batches to help greens wilt, and cook, stirring often, for 8 to 10 more minutes or until greens are tender.

3. Add Savory Sausages, red beans, Spicy Sprinkles, chili powder, oregano, thyme, sea salt, pepper, and hot pepper sauce, and cook, stirring often, for 3 more minutes. Remove from heat. Taste and adjust seasonings as desired, and serve hot.

Variation: You can also serve this over cooked rice or other grains for a one-plate meal. Feel free to replace the collard greens and kale with other greens, such as Swiss chard, turnip greens, or mustard greens.

CORNUCOPIA

Beans and greens are standard fare in the South, and rightfully so. This winning combination is packed with protein, fiber, vitamins, minerals, and phytonutrients. For a full-on down-home meal, serve this dish with pieces of Country Cornbread or Bettermilk Biscuits (recipes in Chapter 5).

Mardi Gras Red Beans

Chewy, crunchy, warm, and spicy, this Mardi Gras–inspired dish is full of fiber, protein, vitamin C, vitamin A, and a batch of phytonutrients that will leave you satisfied with an extra antioxidant boost.

Yield:	Prep time:	Cook time:	Serving size:
7 cups	10 minutes	15 minutes	1½ cups

1 medium yellow onion, diced

½ cup low-sodium vegetable broth

1 large garlic clove, minced

3 medium carrots, diced

3 medium celery stalks, diced

1 large green bell pepper, ribs and seeds removed, and diced

2 (15-oz.) cans red kidney beans or other red beans, drained and rinsed

1 serrano chile pepper, ribs and seeds removed, and finely diced (optional)

1 TB. salt-free Cajun or creole seasoning blend

1 TB. hot pepper sauce

1 TB. chopped fresh parsley

1. In a large pot, combine yellow onion, vegetable broth, and garlic, and sauté over medium heat, stirring often, for 3 to 5 minutes or until onion is soft.

2. Add carrots, celery, and green bell pepper, and cook, stirring often, for 5 more minutes or until vegetables are tender.

3. Stir in kidney beans, serrano chile pepper (if using), Cajun seasoning blend, hot pepper sauce, and parsley. Reduce heat to low, and simmer for 5 minutes or until warmed through. Remove from heat. Serve hot individual servings on a bed of brown or wild rice as desired.

Variation: Not in the mood for Cajun spices? Feel free to replace the Cajun seasoning blend with curry powder for an Indian-flavored dish. Or for **Mexicali Red Beans,** substitute with $\frac{1}{2}$ cup fresh cilantro, 1 teaspoon cocoa powder, 1 teaspoon chili powder, and $\frac{1}{2}$ teaspoon cayenne.

> **MEATLESS AND WHEATLESS**
>
> To make your own salt-free Cajun/creole spice blend, combine 1 teaspoon paprika, 1 teaspoon chili powder, $\frac{3}{4}$ teaspoon dried thyme, $\frac{1}{2}$ teaspoon dried oregano, $\frac{1}{2}$ teaspoon cayenne, $\frac{1}{4}$ teaspoon garlic powder, and $\frac{1}{4}$ teaspoon onion powder. Makes $4\frac{1}{4}$ teaspoons.

Drunken Black Beans

In the Southwest, this dish is traditionally made with pinto beans. To change things up a bit, we've used black beans in our version of this spicy, beer-spiked bean dish.

Yield:	Prep time:	Cook time:	Serving size:
4 or 5 cups	8 to 10 minutes	1 hour	1 cup

4 cups water

1 lb. dried black beans, sorted and rinsed

1 bay leaf

1 (14-oz.) can diced tomatoes with green chiles

1 (12-oz.) bottle gluten-free beer

1 cup yellow onion, diced

1 jalapeño pepper, ribs and seeds removed, and finely diced

2 TB. garlic, minced

2 tsp. dried oregano

1 tsp. ground cumin

$\frac{1}{4}$ cup chopped fresh cilantro

Sea salt

Freshly ground black pepper

1. In a large pot, combine water, black beans, and bay leaf, and bring to a boil over high heat. Cover, reduce heat to low, and simmer, stirring occasionally, for 30 minutes.

2. Stir in diced tomatoes, beer, yellow onion, jalapeño pepper, garlic, oregano, and cumin. Cover and simmer, stirring occasionally, for 30 more minutes or until black beans are tender.

3. Stir in cilantro. Remove from heat, and remove and discard bay leaf. Taste and season with sea salt and pepper as desired. Serve hot with Mexican-style meals or enjoy as a snack with tortilla chips and Whoo-Pea Guacamole (recipe in Chapter 8).

Variation: If you're partial to tequila, replace the beer with ¼ cup tequila. For even more of a kick, add ¼ cup regular or decaf coffee. For an alcohol-free version, replace the beer with 1 cup low-sodium vegetable broth.

CORNUCOPIA

Black beans are commonly referred to as turtle beans, in reference to their shiny, dark, shell-like appearance.

Soy-Catash

Succotash is a traditional side dish often served as part of the Thanksgiving spread in many New England households. Adding shelled edamame bumps up the protein and color contrast of this corn, tomato, and bell pepper creation.

Yield:	Prep time:	Cook time:	Serving size:
4 cups	5 to 7 minutes	10 minutes	1 cup

1½ cups fresh or frozen cut corn kernels

1 cup red bell pepper, diced

½ cup low-sodium vegetable broth

1 cup frozen shelled edamame

1 large Roma tomato, diced

½ cup green onion, thinly sliced

1 tsp. chili powder

½ tsp. sea salt

½ tsp. freshly ground black pepper

¼ cup chopped fresh parsley

1. Place a large, nonstick skillet over medium heat. Add corn, red bell pepper, and vegetable broth, and cook, stirring often, for 5 minutes.

2. Add edamame, Roma tomato, green onion, chili powder, sea salt, and pepper, and cook, stirring often, for 5 more minutes.

3. Stir in parsley. Remove from heat, and serve hot or at room temperature.

Variation: For extra color and contrast, add $\frac{1}{2}$ cup canned kidney beans or black beans. If you can't find shelled edamame, replace it with an equal amount of frozen lima beans.

> **AGAINST THE GRAIN**
>
> You might have seen "non-GMO" on product labels, especially organic ones. GMO is the abbreviation for "genetically modified organism," and this terminology is applied to foods whose genetic material has been altered using high-tech scientific procedures. There's much controversy as to whether this type of technological tampering is harmful to humans, as long-term studies have not been performed. These altering practices are often used with corn and soybean crops, so to be on the safe side, look for "non-GMO" on products that contain these items and opt for organic when it comes to corn and soy products.

Black-Eyed Peas with Cilantro and Leeks

You'll be pleasantly surprised by how well fragrant fresh cilantro and leeks complement the earthy rich black-eyed pea broth. This combo is especially tasty on our Country Cornbread (recipe in Chapter 5).

Yield:	Prep time:	Cook time:	Serving size:
4 or 5 cups	5 to 7 minutes	30 to 40 minutes	1 cup

4 cups water

1 lb. dried black-eyed peas, sorted and rinsed

1 bay leaf

1 leek, cut into quarters lengthwise and thinly sliced

$\frac{1}{2}$ cup low-sodium vegetable broth

$1\frac{1}{2}$ TB. garlic, minced

1 tsp. dried thyme

$\frac{1}{2}$ cup chopped fresh cilantro

Sea salt

Freshly ground black pepper

1. In a large pot, combine water, black-eyed peas, and bay leaf, and bring to a boil over high heat. Cover, reduce heat to low, and simmer, stirring occasionally, for 30 to 40 minutes or until black-eyed peas are tender. Remove and discard bay leaf.

2. Meanwhile, place a large, nonstick skillet over medium heat. Add leek, vegetable broth, garlic, and thyme, and cook, stirring often, for 5 minutes or until leek is soft.

3. When black-eyed peas are tender, add leek mixture and cilantro, and stir well to combine. Remove from heat. Taste and season with sea salt and pepper as desired, and serve hot or at room temperature.

Variation: If you're short on time, you can replace the dried black-eyed pea mixture in step 1 with 2 (15-ounce) cans black-eyed peas, drained and rinsed, add only $\frac{2}{3}$ cup water, omit the bay leaf, and cook the mixture over medium heat, stirring often, for 5 minutes.

CORNUCOPIA

Depending on the region, black-eyed peas are also known by quite a few other names, such as cowpeas, crowder peas, Southern beans/peas, or cream peas. Eating black-eyed peas on New Year's Day is thought to bring prosperity, and who couldn't use some more of that?

French-Style Peas with Smoky Tempeh Un-Bacon

Sweet peas and red onion combine with pieces of our Smoky Tempeh Un-Bacon and what may seem like a surprising ingredient—savoy cabbage. This dish is inspired by a classic French recipe, which typically features tender lettuce leaves.

Yield:	Prep time:	Cook time:	Serving size:
4 cups	5 to 7 minutes	7 to 12 minutes	1 cup

1 cup red onion, cut into half moons

4 slices Smoky Tempeh Un-Bacon (recipe in Chapter 12), cut into $\frac{1}{2}$-in. pieces

1 TB. olive oil

1 (16-oz.) pkg. frozen peas

$\frac{1}{2}$ cup low-sodium vegetable broth or water

$\frac{1}{2}$ tsp. dried dill weed

$\frac{1}{2}$ tsp. sea salt

$\frac{1}{4}$ tsp. freshly ground black pepper

$1\frac{1}{2}$ cups savoy cabbage, roughly chopped

$\frac{1}{4}$ cup chopped fresh parsley

1. In a large, nonstick skillet, combine red onion, Smoky Tempeh Un-Bacon, and olive oil, and sauté over medium heat, stirring often, for 3 to 5 minutes or until red onion is soft and bacon is crispy.

2. Add peas, vegetable broth, dill weed, sea salt, and pepper, and cook, stirring often, for 3 to 5 more minutes or until peas are tender and bright green.

3. Add savoy cabbage and parsley, and cook, stirring often, for 1 or 2 more minutes or until cabbage begins to wilt. Remove from heat, and serve hot.

Variation: If you prefer to make this recipe in the traditional manner, replace the savoy cabbage with Boston lettuce and the red onion with whole pearl onions. You can also add $\frac{1}{2}$ cup diced red bell pepper for extra flavor and color.

Plant-Based Dietitian Recommends: Substitute an additional $\frac{1}{4}$ cup vegetable broth or water for the oil for a total of $\frac{3}{4}$ cup for the whole recipe.

MEATLESS AND WHEATLESS

In many recipes, we call for "onion, cut into half moons." Here's how you do that: cut the peeled onion in half, from the top to the root end. Place the cut side down, and vertically cut thin slices from the top to the root end.

Green Beans Amandine

Garnishing tender cooked green beans with almonds, or *amandine* style, provides a bit of crunchiness, and the addition of slightly smoky, toasted sesame oil deepens the almonds' subtle flavor.

Yield:	Prep time:	Cook time:	Serving size:
4 cups	5 minutes	8 to 12 minutes	1 cup

½ cup raw sliced almonds or whole almonds, roughly chopped

1 (16-oz.) pkg. frozen whole green beans or 1 lb. fresh green beans, cut into 4-in. pieces

½ cup low-sodium vegetable broth or water

1 TB. garlic, minced

3 TB. chopped fresh parsley

1 TB. wheat-free tamari or Bragg Liquid Aminos

½ TB. toasted sesame oil

½ tsp. freshly ground black pepper or garlic pepper

1. In a large, nonstick skillet, place almonds, and cook over medium heat, shaking skillet often, for 3 to 5 minutes or until lightly toasted and fragrant. Transfer almonds to a small bowl, and set aside.

2. Return the skillet to medium heat. Add green beans, vegetable broth, and garlic, and cook, stirring often, for 5 to 7 minutes or until green beans are crisp-tender.

3. Add parsley, tamari, toasted sesame oil, and pepper, and stir well. Remove from heat, and serve hot or at room temperature as desired.

Variation: For added color and flavor, add ½ cup julienned red bell pepper and 1 tablespoon minced fresh ginger.

Plant-Based Dietitian Recommends: Omit the oil.

> **DEFINITION**
>
> *Amandine* is a French culinary term that indicates the final dish has a garnish of whole, sliced, or toasted almonds. In many American cookbooks, this term is often erroneously spelled as *almondine*. Plant-based dishes frequently served amandine style include asparagus, green beans, and potatoes.

BBQ Baked Beans

In this authentic slow-cooked version of baked beans, freshly cooked navy beans are flavored with sweet sorghum, maple syrup, and our zesty and boozy Bourbon Blues BBQ Sauce.

Yield:	Prep time:	Cook time:	Serving size:
8 or 9 cups	10 minutes	2 to 2½ hours	1 cup

6 cups water

1 lb. dried navy beans, sorted and rinsed

1 bay leaf

2 cups yellow onion, diced

⅔ cup low-sodium vegetable broth

2 TB. garlic, minced

½ cup Bourbon Blues BBQ Sauce (recipe in Chapter 9)

3 TB. maple syrup

2 TB. sorghum syrup

1 TB. spicy brown mustard

1 tsp. sea salt

½ tsp. freshly ground black pepper

1. In a large pot, combine water, navy beans, and bay leaf, and bring to a boil over high heat. Cover, reduce heat to low, and simmer for 1 to 1½ hours or until navy beans are tender. Remove from heat, and remove and discard bay leaf.

2. Meanwhile, place a medium, nonstick skillet over medium heat. Add yellow onion, vegetable broth, and garlic, and cook, stirring often, for 5 minutes or until onions are soft. Remove from heat.

3. Preheat the oven to 300°F.

4. Transfer cooked navy beans and remaining cooking liquid to a 2½-quart baking dish. Add onion mixture, Bourbon Blues BBQ Sauce, maple syrup, sorghum syrup, spicy brown mustard, sea salt, and pepper, and stir well. Cover baking dish with a lid or a layer of parchment paper and aluminum foil, and bake for 30 minutes. Remove from the oven, and serve hot or at room temperature as desired.

Variation: For even more flavor, add 4 slices Smoky Tempeh Un-Bacon (recipe in Chapter 12), chopped, to the cooked onion mixture.

CORNUCOPIA

In the early 1900s, molasses production was a major industry for Boston, and naturally, this sticky and sweet syrup found its way into many of the city's favorite dishes, including their famous molasses-enhanced Boston Baked Beans. Thus Boston became Beantown.

A Little Something on the Side

In This Chapter

- Stovetop stars
- Oven-baked sides
- Hearty stuffing
- Sensational stuffed squash

We love vegetables! Boiled, broiled, steamed, simmered, stir-fried, grilled, quickly baked, or slowly roasted—put them in front of us, and we'll devour them. In this chapter, you'll find recipes for everything from mashed potatoes to glazed sweet potatoes, cornbread stuffing, and even a grain and dried fruit–stuffed squash that could work as an entrée. And most of these recipes are perfect to carry to a potluck so you know you'll have something yummy to eat!

How thick or thin and small or large you cut your veggies determines how long they take to cook. If you're in a hurry, slice them into thin or small pieces, and stir-fry them in a little vegetable broth or oil; add in some of your favorite fresh or dried herbs, spices, and other seasonings; and in no time, you have one heck of a side dish. Or combine a few of our offerings in this chapter for a veggie-packed meal.

Sizzling Stir-Fried Veggies

Asian flavors of ginger, tamari, and red pepper flakes meld with sweet apricot preserves to spice up this colorful and sweet combination of crunchy vegetables.

Yield:	Prep time:	Cook time:	Serving size:
8 cups	10 to 15 minutes	10 to 15 minutes	1½ cups

2 cups yellow onion, diced

1¾ cups red bell pepper, diced

3 cups shiitake mushrooms, thinly sliced

2 TB. low-sodium vegetable broth or water

½ cup wheat-free tamari or Bragg Liquid Aminos

6 TB. unsweetened apricot preserves

2 TB. brown rice vinegar

2 TB. cornstarch

1 TB. fresh ginger, minced

1 TB. garlic, minced

2 tsp. crushed red pepper flakes

5 cups napa cabbage, roughly chopped

5 cups broccoli florets

1½ cups snow peas, stems removed

2 TB. gomasio

1. In a large *wok*, combine yellow onion, red bell pepper, shiitake mushrooms, and vegetable broth, and sauté over medium-high heat, stirring often with tongs, for 3 to 5 minutes or until vegetables are soft.

2. Meanwhile, in a medium bowl, whisk together tamari, apricot preserves, brown rice vinegar, cornstarch, ginger, garlic, and crushed red pepper flakes, and set aside.

3. To the wok, add napa cabbage, broccoli, and snow peas, and continue to cook, stirring often, for 2 more minutes.

4. Pour sauce mixture on top of vegetables, stir well to combine, and cook for 2 or 3 more minutes. Sprinkle gomasio over top. Remove from heat, and serve hot, alone or over brown rice noodles, brown rice, or quinoa as desired.

Variation: You can also add 1 cup roughly chopped Miso-Glazed Tofu (recipe in Chapter 12) or chopped tempeh. Substitute equal amounts of any vegetables you have in your refrigerator.

Southern Smothered Greens

Get ready for a tasty pot of your favorite greens, cooked up Southern-style with onion, garlic, and seasonings, which yield plenty of *pot liquor* for your enjoyment.

Yield:	Prep time:	Cook time:	Serving size:
6 cups	7 to 10 minutes	20 to 25 minutes	¾ to 1 cup

2 Savory Sausages (recipe in Chapter 12), cut in half lengthwise and thinly sliced

1 cup yellow onion, diced

3 TB. garlic, minced

1 TB. olive oil

1½ cups low-sodium vegetable broth or water

1½ tsp. dried thyme

2 bunches collard greens, turnip greens, kale, Swiss chard, or a combination of greens, washed well, stems removed or trimmed, and torn or cut into large bite-size pieces

1½ TB. nutritional yeast flakes

1 TB. wheat-free tamari

½ tsp. freshly ground black pepper

½ tsp. crushed red pepper flakes or hot pepper sauce

1. Place a large pot over medium heat. Add Savory Sausages, yellow onion, garlic, and olive oil, and sauté, stirring often, for 5 minutes.

2. Add vegetable broth and thyme, and bring to a boil. In batches, add collard greens, covering pot between batches to help greens wilt, and cook, stirring often, for 20 to 25 more minutes or until greens are very tender.

3. Stir in nutritional yeast flakes, tamari, pepper, and crushed red pepper flakes. Remove from heat, and serve hot.

Variation: Feel free to also add ½ cup diced green or red bell pepper to the sautéing onion mixture, or 1 cup canned beans to the finished greens.

Plant-Based Dietitian Recommends: Substitute 2 or 3 tablespoons vegetable broth or water for olive oil.

> **DEFINITION**
>
> **Pot liquor** (a.k.a. pot likker) is the term used to affectionately describe the flavorful and nutritious liquid that accumulates from cooking vegetables, most notably green leafy vegetables. So don't discard it! It's customary to sop up your pot liquor with pieces of bread, cornbread, or biscuits, so check out Chapter 5 for our recipes for all these.

Mmm Mmm Mashed Potatoes

Buttery Yukon gold potatoes are the best choice for making a great-tasting batch of mashed potatoes. To heighten their flavor and creamy texture, we mash them up with some roasted garlic and soy milk.

Yield:	Prep time:	Cook time:	Serving size:
6 cups	10 to 15 minutes	15 to 20 minutes	1 cup

8 to 10 large garlic cloves, peeled

3 lb. (about 8 cups) Yukon gold potatoes, peeled and cut into 2-in. pieces

$\frac{1}{2}$ cup soy milk or other nondairy milk

$\frac{1}{2}$ cup low-sodium vegetable broth

2 TB. nutritional yeast flakes

$1\frac{1}{2}$ TB. nonhydrogenated margarine (optional)

1 tsp. sea salt

$\frac{1}{2}$ tsp. freshly ground black pepper, white pepper, or garlic pepper

1. Preheat the oven to 375°F.

2. Cut a 6-inch-square piece of parchment paper and aluminum foil. Place the parchment paper on top of the aluminum foil. Place garlic cloves in the center of the parchment paper, and fold over edges of the paper to enclose them. Gather the corners of the aluminum foil, crimp to enclose the parchment paper, and place the packet in a pie pan.

3. Bake for 10 to 15 minutes or until garlic in the packet feels soft when gently squeezed. Remove from the oven, and let cool for 5 minutes.

4. Meanwhile, place Yukon gold potatoes in a large pot, cover with water, and cook over medium-high heat for 15 to 20 minutes or until potatoes are tender. Remove from heat. Reserve 1 cup cooking liquid, drain potatoes in a colander, and return potatoes to the pot.

5. In a small bowl, mash garlic cloves with a fork to form a smooth paste.

6. Add mashed garlic cloves, soy milk, vegetable broth, nutritional yeast flakes, margarine (if using), sea salt, and pepper to the pot, and either mash with a potato masher or beat with an electric mixer on medium speed for 2 or 3 minutes or until potatoes are as smooth as desired. Add a little reserved cooking liquid as needed to achieve desired consistency. Serve hot, alone, topped with Roasted Onion and Garlic Gravy (recipe in Chapter 9), or use as desired in your favorite recipes.

Variation: Vary the flavor by stirring in 1 or 2 tablespoons wasabi powder, $\frac{1}{3}$ cup sun-dried tomato pieces, or $\frac{1}{2}$ cup shredded Mellow Jack Cheese or Better Cheddar (recipes in Chapter 6).

Plant-Based Dietitian Recommends: Omit the optional margarine.

MEATLESS AND WHEATLESS

Roasted garlic cloves are a very versatile ingredient for adding a bit of extra flavor to a recipe. You can slice them and add to sauces, cooked grains, and veggie side dishes, or blend them in salad dressings. One of the best and easiest ways to enjoy them is to spread a clove or two on a slice of bread.

Maple-Glazed Sweet Potatoes

We infuse our sweet potatoes by cooking them in a lightly spiced apple juice mixture, glaze them with a little maple syrup, and finish with a sprinkling of crunchy toasted pecans over the top. The perfect fall and winter holiday dish.

Yield:	Prep time:	Cook time:	Serving size:
6 cups	5 to 7 minutes	20 to 25 minutes	1 cup

3 lb. (about 8 cups) sweet potatoes, cut into 2-in. cubes

⅔ cup apple juice or water

1¼ tsp. ground cinnamon

¾ tsp. ground ginger

½ cup raw pecan pieces

⅓ cup maple syrup

Sea salt

1. In a large, nonstick skillet, combine sweet potatoes, apple juice, cinnamon, and ginger, and bring to a boil over high heat. Cover, reduce heat to medium, and cook for 15 to 20 minutes or until sweet potatoes are tender.

2. Meanwhile, in a small, nonstick skillet, place pecans, and cook over medium heat, shaking the skillet often, for 3 to 5 minutes or until lightly toasted and fragrant. Transfer pecans to a small bowl, and set aside.

3. When sweet potatoes are tender, stir in maple syrup, and cook, stirring occasionally, for 2 more minutes. Taste and season with sea salt as desired. Sprinkle toasted pecans over the top, remove from heat, and serve hot or at room temperature as desired.

Variation: Feel free to replace the sweet potatoes with garnet yams. For an even more flavorful dish, replace the apple juice with spiced apple cider.

AGAINST THE GRAIN

Nuts and seeds are rich in essential fatty acids that are good for your health, but this natural fat content can also cause them to turn rancid quite quickly. To extend their shelf life, store raw nuts and seeds in airtight containers in the refrigerator or freezer. Also, for the best prices, purchase them from the bulk bins of your local grocery or natural foods store rather than packaged.

Two-Potato Fries

These healthy fries, made with generously seasoned russets and sweet potatoes, are baked instead of fried.

Yield:	Prep time:	Cook time:	Serving size:
6 cups	5 to 7 minutes	35 to 40 minutes	1 cup

3 cups (1 or 2 large potatoes) russet potatoes, cut into 3×½-in.-thick french fries

3 cups (1 or 2 large potatoes) sweet potatoes, cut into 3×½-in.-thick french fries

2 TB. low-sodium vegetable broth

1½ TB. olive oil

1 TB. nutritional yeast flakes or Italian Herb Sprinkles (variation in Chapter 6)

1½ tsp. dried basil

1 tsp. garlic powder or garlic granules

1 tsp. onion powder

1 tsp. chili powder

¾ tsp. sea salt

½ tsp. freshly ground black pepper

1. Preheat the oven to 425°F. Line a cookie sheet with parchment paper or a Silpat liner.

2. In a large bowl, combine russet potatoes, sweet potatoes, vegetable broth, olive oil, nutritional yeast flakes, basil, garlic powder, onion powder, chili powder, sea salt, and pepper. Using your hands, toss mixture until evenly coated.

3. Transfer mixture to the prepared cookie sheet, and spread out to form a single layer. Bake for 20 minutes.

4. Remove from the oven, stir with a spatula, and spread out into a single layer again. Bake for 15 to 20 more minutes or until desired doneness. Remove from the oven, and serve hot.

Variation: For slightly different herb-flavored fries, replace the dried basil with 1 tablespoon herbes de Provence.

Plant-Based Dietitian Recommends: Substitute an extra 3 tablespoons vegetable broth for the oil (for a total of 5 tablespoons broth).

> **CORNUCOPIA**
>
> The most popular vegetable side dish in the United States is french fries. Unfortunately, most of them are deep-fried from fast-food restaurants, where each serving is high in fat, calories, and sodium. However with these baked Two-Potato Fries, you still get to enjoy great-tasting fries, but without the unnecessary dietary pitfalls.

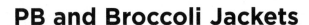

PB and Broccoli Jackets

You might not think baked potatoes and peanut butter are a natural combination … until you taste it! We bet you'll love this baked potato with healthy, hearty fillings and a spicy peanut butter sauce.

Yield:	Prep time:	Cook time:	Serving size:
6 potatoes	15 minutes	30 to 45 minutes	1 potato

6 russet potatoes	$\frac{1}{3}$ cup cilantro leaves
6 cups broccoli florets	$\frac{1}{4}$ cup brown rice vinegar
$\frac{1}{2}$ cup wheat-free tamari or Bragg Liquid Aminos	$\frac{1}{4}$ cup maple syrup
$\frac{1}{2}$ cup natural peanut butter	1 TB. garlic, minced
$\frac{1}{2}$ cup warm water	1 TB. fresh ginger, minced
	1 TB. crushed red pepper flakes

1. Preheat the oven to 350°F.

2. Wash and wrap russet potatoes in a layer of parchment paper, covered by a layer of aluminum foil. Place on a cookie sheet, and bake for 30 minutes or until soft. Remove from the oven, and set aside.

3. Place a steamer basket in a medium pot, add several inches of water, and bring to a boil over medium-high heat. Place broccoli in the steamer basket and allow to steam for 5 to 8 minutes or until crisp-tender.

4. Meanwhile, in a blender, combine tamari, peanut butter, warm water, cilantro, brown rice vinegar, maple syrup, garlic, ginger, and crushed red pepper flakes, and blend for 1 minute or until smooth.

5. Cut each potato in half lengthwise, and spoon 1 cup steamed broccoli on top of each potato. Pour approximately $\frac{1}{3}$ cup peanut butter sauce evenly onto each potato, and serve warm.

Variation: Feel free to use sweet potatoes or yams instead of russet potatoes and cauliflower instead of broccoli.

> **MEATLESS AND WHEATLESS**
>
> You can use this spicy peanut butter sauce on top of any vegetable, whole grain, or pasta. It even tastes delicious as a salad dressing.

Colorific Cauliflower and Broccoli Gratin

A *gratin* is French for both an oven-proof baking dish as well as a casserole topped with a breadcrumb mixture, and this recipe is just that. It's made with broccoli and two different colored cauliflowers all covered in a crunchy topping.

Yield:	Prep time:	Cook time:	Serving size:
8 cups	10 to 15 minutes	30 to 35 minutes	1 cup

2 cups broccoli florets

2 cups cauliflower florets

2 cups orange or purple cauliflower florets

$\frac{1}{3}$ cup low-sodium vegetable broth

3 TB. Italian Herb Sprinkles (variation in Chapter 6) or nutritional yeast flakes

1 tsp. garlic powder or garlic granules

Sea salt

Freshly ground black pepper

2 slices Multi-Grain Sandwich Bread (recipe in Chapter 5)

$\frac{1}{2}$ cup shredded Mellow Jack Cheese or Better Cheddar (recipes in Chapter 6)

2 TB. chopped fresh parsley

1 TB. Italian seasoning blend or 1 tsp. each dried basil, oregano, and thyme

1. Preheat the oven to 375°F. Lightly oil a 9×13-inch baking pan.

2. In a large bowl, combine broccoli, cauliflower, orange cauliflower, vegetable broth, $1\frac{1}{2}$ tablespoons Italian Herb Sprinkles, and $\frac{1}{2}$ teaspoon garlic powder. Season with sea salt and pepper as desired, and stir well to combine. Transfer broccoli-cauliflower mixture to the prepared baking pan.

3. In a food processor fitted with an S blade, place slices of Multi-Grain Sandwich Bread, and process for 1 minute or until you get fine crumbs. Measure out 1 cup breadcrumbs (save any extra for use in another recipe), and transfer breadcrumbs to a small bowl.

4. Add Mellow Jack Cheese, parsley, Italian seasoning blend, remaining $1\frac{1}{2}$ tablespoons Italian Herb Sprinkles, and remaining $\frac{1}{2}$ teaspoon garlic powder, and stir well to combine.

5. Evenly sprinkle breadcrumb mixture over broccoli-cauliflower mixture. Bake for 30 to 35 minutes or until vegetables are tender and breadcrumbs are golden brown.

Variation: For an even more colorful gratin, replace 2 cups broccoli with 2 cups broccoli romanesco, cut into florets, and omit the white cauliflower and only use orange and purple cauliflower. To transform this dish into **Cauliflower and Broccoli Au Gratin,** steam or blanch the broccoli and cauliflower until crisp-tender. Transfer to a casserole dish, along with the other vegetable broth mixture ingredients, and add either 2 cups Béchamel Sauce (recipe in Chapter 9) and an additional 1 cup shredded Mellow Jack Cheese (or Better Cheddar), or combine them with $1\frac{1}{2}$ cups Cheesy Sauce (recipe in Chapter 6) and 1 cup soy milk (or water). Top either version with breadcrumb mixture and bake as directed.

CORNUCOPIA

Most people are familiar with the bright white heads of cauliflower, but it's also available in other colors, like purple, orange, and pale green as its closely related cousins broccoflower or the spectacular spiked variation broccoli romanesco. You can often find these colorful cruciferous veggies in the produce section of your local grocery and natural foods stores and at farmers' markets.

Festive Stuffed Squash

Small *carnival squashes* are stuffed with a mixture of quinoa, wild rice, savory aromatic vegetables, dried fruit, and nuts, and baked until soft.

Yield:	Prep time:	Cook time:	Serving size:
6 squashes	20 to 25 minutes	60 to 70 minutes	1 squash

½ cup raw pecan pieces

1 cup crimini mushrooms, cut in half and thinly sliced

⅔ cup red onion, diced

⅔ cup celery, diced

2 tsp. olive oil

½ cup green onion, thinly sliced

2 TB. garlic, minced

1½ TB. chopped fresh thyme or 1½ tsp. dried thyme

1 TB. chopped fresh sage or 1 tsp. rubbed sage

½ tsp. sea salt

½ tsp. freshly ground black pepper or garlic pepper

2¼ cups low-sodium vegetable broth

¾ cup wild rice

1 cup quinoa

1¾ cups water

6 medium carnival squash (about 1 lb. each)

½ cup dried cherries or roughly chopped pitted dates

½ cup dried cranberries

½ cup dried apricots, thinly sliced

⅓ cup chopped fresh parsley

1. In a large saucepan, place pecans, and cook over medium heat, shaking the saucepan often, for 3 to 5 minutes or until lightly toasted and fragrant. Transfer pecans to a small bowl, and set aside.

2. Return the saucepan to medium heat. Add crimini mushrooms, red onion, celery, and olive oil, and sauté, stirring often, for 5 minutes.

3. Add green onion, garlic, thyme, sage, sea salt, and pepper, and sauté, stirring often, for 2 more minutes.

4. Add vegetable broth and wild rice, increase heat to high, and bring to a boil. Cover, reduce heat to low, and simmer for 40 minutes or until wild rice is tender and all liquid is absorbed. Remove from heat.

5. Place quinoa in a fine mesh sieve, and rinse well under running water for 1 minute. In a small saucepan, combine water and quinoa, and bring to a boil over high heat. Cover, reduce heat to low, and simmer for 18 to 20 minutes or until quinoa is tender and all liquid is absorbed. Remove from heat.

6. Preheat the oven to 350°F.

7. While grains are cooking, prep carnival squashes. Using a sharp knife, cut off top of each squash, 1 inch down from stem end. Using a spoon, scoop out and discard seeds. If needed, shave a little off the bottom of each squash so it stands upright. Place squashes side by side and upright in a large baking dish, and bake for 25 minutes.

8. Fluff wild rice mixture and quinoa with a fork to loosen grains. Add quinoa to wild rice mixture along with dried cherries, dried cranberries, dried apricots, and parsley, and stir gently to combine.

9. Remove baked squashes from the oven. Evenly divide wild rice mixture among squashes. Return squashes to the oven and bake for 20 to 25 more minutes or until squashes are tender. Remove from the oven, and serve hot.

Variation: Feel free to replace the carnival squash with acorn, delicate, sweet dumpling, or other winter squash. You can also replace the pecans with other roughly chopped nuts, such as walnuts, almonds, or hazelnuts, and the dried fruits we've suggested can be replaced with raisins, currants, apples, peaches, etc.

Plant-Based Dietitian Recommends: Substitute an additional 2 or 3 tablespoons vegetable broth or water for olive oil.

> **DEFINITION**
>
> **Carnival squash** are small pumpkin-shape squashes and come in several shades, such as pale yellow to cream, with orange, pale, or dark-green spots or vertical stripes. They're similar in flavor to sweet potato or butternut squash and are quite delish when baked, steamed, puréed, or used in soups and stews.

Cornbread Stuffing

Using our golden Country Cornbread, aromatic vegetables, and some fresh herbs, you can mix up a batch of this flavorful stuffing that's sure to be a welcome addition to any meal.

Yield:	Prep time:	Cook time:	Serving size:
8 or 9 cups	15 minutes, plus 1 hour dry time	30 to 40 minutes	1 cup

1 (9-in.) Country Cornbread (recipe in Chapter 5)

1$\frac{1}{2}$ cups yellow onion, diced

1$\frac{1}{2}$ cups celery, diced

1 TB. olive oil

1 cup green onion, thinly sliced

2 TB. garlic, minced

2 TB. chopped fresh thyme or 2 tsp. dried thyme

1$\frac{1}{2}$ TB. chopped fresh sage or 1$\frac{1}{2}$ tsp. rubbed sage

1 tsp. chili powder

$\frac{1}{2}$ cup chopped fresh parsley (preferably Italian flat-leaf parsley)

2 TB. nutritional yeast flakes

$\frac{1}{2}$ tsp. sea salt

$\frac{1}{2}$ tsp. freshly ground black pepper or garlic pepper

$\frac{2}{3}$ to $\frac{3}{4}$ cup low-sodium vegetable broth

1. Prepare Country Cornbread according to the recipe instructions, at least 1 day ahead (or more) to allow it to dry out a bit. Cut it into 1-inch cubes, place cubes on a cookie sheet, and set aside for 1 hour to allow cubes to dry out even more.

2. Preheat the oven to 350°F. Lightly oil a 9×13-inch baking pan or a large casserole dish.

3. While cornbread cubes are drying out, place a large, nonstick skillet over medium heat. Add yellow onion, celery, and olive oil, and sauté, stirring often, for 5 minutes.

4. Add green onion, garlic, thyme, sage, and chili powder, and sauté, stirring often, for 2 more minutes. Remove from heat.

5. Transfer cornbread cubes to a large bowl. Add sautéed onion mixture, parsley, nutritional yeast flakes, sea salt, and pepper, and toss gently to combine. Add enough vegetable broth to moisten cornbread stuffing mixture, but don't make it soggy. Taste and adjust seasonings as desired.

6. Transfer cornbread stuffing mixture to the prepared pan. Cover with a lid or a layer of parchment paper and aluminum foil, and bake for 25 minutes. If you like the top of your stuffing crispy, remove the lid (or parchment paper and aluminum foil) and bake for 5 to 10 more minutes or until lightly browned on top. Remove from the oven, and serve hot.

Variation: For even more flavor, add 4 slices Smoky Tempeh Un-Bacon, chopped, or 2 chopped Savory Sausages (recipes in Chapter 12) to the sautéed onion mixture. For a more traditional **Bread Stuffing**, replace the Country Cornbread with 1 loaf Multi-Grain Sandwich Bread, cut into 1-inch cubes (about 8 or 9 cups bread cubes), plus an additional $\frac{1}{2}$ to $\frac{2}{3}$ cup vegetable broth as needed.

Plant-Based Dietitian Recommends: Substitute 2 or 3 tablespoons vegetable broth or water for olive oil.

MEATLESS AND WHEATLESS

Whether you call them green onions, spring onions, or scallions, they're all the same. These mild-flavored alliums, sold bundled together in bunches, are great for adding a bit of oniony flavor and color to your favorite dishes.

Divine Desserts

Welcome to your very own gluten-free vegan bake shop! In Part 6, you learn how to make many of the sweet treats you thought you would no longer be able to have since going gluten free and vegan, plus a few new ones you may have never thought possible. So tie on your prettiest apron, gather up your baking supplies, and stock up your pantry and fridge with all the gluten-free vegan staples you learned about in Chapter 2. Then flip through the chapters in this part, find a recipe that suits your mood or craving, and get ready to bake some scrumptiously celestial desserts in your kitchen!

Forget eggs and the dairy case. You don't need either, and you won't miss them. In the following chapters, you learn how easy it is to create tantalizing sweet treats such as crisp and chewy cookies, moist brownies, and fruit-filled pies and tarts. We also give you an amazing collection of cakes, cakelike creations, and even creamy cheesecake.

And for those of you who are currently using your oven for storage rather than baking, you'll hurry to clean it out when you see the recipes for layered fruit parfaits, rich-tasting dessert toppings, creamy mousse, and comforting tapioca pudding.

Okay, we've teased you enough. Get to it, and create your own divine desserts that are all gluten free, vegan, and totally delicious!

From the Cookie Jar

In This Chapter

- Cut-and-roll cookies
- Scoop-and-smash cookies
- Brownies and no-bake bars

For many of us, the simple act of making a batch of cookies brings back fond memories of times spent with mothers and grandmothers, mixing batters and baking cookies. Hopefully, by preparing one or more of the recipes in this chapter, you'll be able to rekindle your love affair with from-scratch baking, and maybe even begin new traditions of gluten-free vegan baking with those near and dear to you.

We start off this chapter's recipes with classic, slightly sweet, cut-out cookies. Enjoy them plain, or decorate them to your heart's desire. We also offer gluten-free and vegan revamps of other traditional cookies, like snickerdoodles, peanut butter, and chocolate chip. And last but not least, we've included recipes for making your own chocolaty brownies and energy bars. It's time to bake up a batch of cookies to fill up your cookie jar!

Plant-Based Dietitian Recommends: The recipes in this chapter should be considered special treats, especially if you have a health issue or are trying to lose weight. Opt for choices like the Fudgy Brownies and Crispy Rice Trail Mix Bars to indulge in occasionally.

Cut-Out Cookies

It's time to bust out your cookie cutters! These slightly sweet cookies are perfect for all your holiday needs or even for enjoying on an average weekday.

Yield:	Prep time:	Cook time:	Serving size:
3 or 4 dozen cookies (depending on size)	10 minutes, plus 1 hour chill time	8 to 10 minutes	2 cookies

$^2/_3$ cup nonhydrogenated margarine	$2^1/_4$ cups Bob's Red Mill Gluten-Free All-Purpose Baking Flour
$^1/_2$ cup unbleached cane sugar	$^1/_2$ cup tapioca starch
$1^1/_2$ tsp. alcohol-free vanilla extract	$^1/_2$ tsp. gluten-free xanthan gum
	$^1/_4$ tsp. sea salt

1. In a large bowl, combine margarine, unbleached cane sugar, and vanilla extract until light and creamy.

2. Add Bob's Red Mill Gluten-Free All-Purpose Baking Flour, tapioca starch, xanthan gum, and sea salt, and stir well until mixture forms a soft dough. Cover and chill for 1 hour or until firm.

3. Preheat the oven to 350°F.

4. Divide cookie dough in half. Work with only one half at a time, and keep remaining dough covered. Place half of dough between 2 (12×16-inch) pieces of parchment paper or Silpat liners. Using a rolling pin, roll out dough to desired thickness ($^1/_8$ inch thick for crispy cookies or $^1/_4$ inch thick for soft cookies).

5. Peel off top sheet of parchment paper or remove top Silpat liner. Cut into shapes with cookie cutters (or a knife) as desired, leaving a 1-inch space between cookies. Carefully transfer parchment paper to a cookie sheet. Leave cookies plain or sprinkle with a little additional unbleached cane sugar before baking, or decorate with frosting after baking as desired.

6. Repeat rolling and cutting procedure with remaining cookie dough. Gather up scraps from each half, and repeat rolling and cutting procedure as needed.

7. Bake for 8 to 10 minutes or until very lightly browned on the bottom. Remove from the oven. Let cool slightly before transferring cookies to a rack to cool completely. Store cookies in an airtight container at room temperature.

Variation: For crisper, white **Arrowroot Cookies,** replace the Gluten-Free All-Purpose Baking Flour with Beverly's Baking Blend (recipe in Chapter 3) and the tapioca starch with arrowroot. To make lemon-, lime-, or orange-flavored **Citrus Cut-Out Cookies,** omit the vanilla extract and add 2 tablespoons freshly squeezed citrus juice and 1 teaspoon zest. For **Chocolate Cut-Out Cookies,** use only $\frac{1}{3}$ cup tapioca starch and add $\frac{1}{4}$ cup cocoa powder.

> **MEATLESS AND WHEATLESS**
>
> If you'd like to decorate your baked cookies with frosting, stir together 1 cup vegan confectioners' sugar, $\frac{1}{2}$ teaspoon vanilla extract, and add 1 teaspoon non-dairy milk (your choice) at a time until desired consistency. To naturally tint your frosting, replace the nondairy milk with grape, raspberry, or cherry juice, or add a pinch of turmeric (for yellow) or spirulina or blue-green algae powder (for green).

Snickerdoodles

The smell of these cinnamon-sugar-coated cookies baking will permeate your house and have you eagerly awaiting your first bite. But be patient and let them cool sufficiently so they don't crumble.

Yield:	Prep time:	Cook time:	Serving size:
$2\frac{1}{2}$ to 3 dozen cookies	10 to 12 minutes	12 to 14 minutes	2 cookies

2 TB. plus 1 cup unbleached cane sugar

2 tsp. ground cinnamon

6 TB. water

2 TB. ground *golden flaxseeds* or flaxseed meal

6 TB. nonhydrogenated margarine

$1\frac{1}{2}$ tsp. alcohol-free vanilla extract

$2\frac{2}{3}$ cups Bob's Red Mill Gluten-Free All-Purpose Baking Flour

$\frac{1}{2}$ cup arrowroot

$\frac{3}{4}$ tsp. baking soda

$\frac{3}{4}$ tsp. gluten-free xanthan gum

$\frac{1}{4}$ tsp. sea salt

1. Preheat the oven to 350°F. Line 2 large cookie sheets with parchment paper or Silpat liners.

2. In a small bowl, combine 2 tablespoons unbleached cane sugar and cinnamon, and set aside.

3. In a large bowl, combine water and golden flaxseeds, and let sit for 5 minutes. Add remaining 1 cup unbleached cane sugar, margarine, and vanilla extract, and stir together until light and creamy.

4. Add Bob's Red Mill Gluten-Free All-Purpose Baking Flour, arrowroot, baking soda, xanthan gum, and sea salt, and stir well until mixture forms a soft dough.

5. Using your hands, roll cookie dough into 1½-inch balls. Roll each ball in cinnamon-sugar mixture, and place cookies on the prepared cookie sheets, spacing them 2 inches apart. Using a flat-bottomed glass, gently and slightly flatten each ball.

6. Bake for 12 to 14 minutes or until very lightly browned on the bottom. Remove from the oven. Let cool slightly before transferring cookies to a rack to cool completely. Store cookies in an airtight container at room temperature.

Variation: For dome-shape snickerdoodles, don't flatten the cookie dough balls prior to baking.

DEFINITION

Golden flaxseeds are the pale yellow sister of the more commonly used nutty brown flaxseeds. Both forms of flaxseeds can be used interchangeably on foods and in recipes. But because they're lighter in color, the golden flaxseeds are less visible in baked goods, which can be preferable in light-colored cookie and cake batters.

Peanut Butter Cookies

Using two kinds of sugar in these cookies helps keep them moist yet chewy, and the ground flaxseeds help bind the cookie batter and accentuate the peanut butter flavor.

Yield:	Prep time:	Cook time:	Serving size:
2½ to 3 dozen cookies	10 minutes	12 to 14 minutes	2 cookies

5 TB. water

2 TB. ground flaxseeds or flaxseed meal

1 tsp. plus ½ cup unbleached cane sugar

½ cup turbinado sugar or vegan light brown sugar

½ cup natural peanut butter

¼ cup sunflower oil or other oil

1 tsp. alcohol-free vanilla extract

2 cups Beverly's Baking Blend (recipe in Chapter 3)

1 tsp. gluten-free xanthan gum

½ tsp. baking soda

½ tsp. sea salt

1. Preheat the oven to 350°F. Line 2 large cookie sheets with parchment paper or Silpat liners.

2. In a large bowl, combine water and flaxseeds, and let sit for 5 minutes.

3. In a small bowl, place 1 teaspoon unbleached cane sugar, and set aside.

4. To flaxseed mixture, add remaining ½ cup unbleached cane sugar, turbinado sugar, peanut butter, sunflower oil, and vanilla extract, and stir together until light and creamy.

5. Add Beverly's Baking Blend, xanthan gum, baking soda, and sea salt, and stir well until mixture forms a soft dough.

6. Portion cookie dough using a 2-inch scoop or heaping 2 tablespoonfuls onto the prepared cookie sheets, spacing them 2 inches apart. Using the tines of a fork dipped into the reserved unbleached sugar, flatten each cookie slightly in a criss-cross pattern. Then sprinkle a pinch of unbleached cane sugar over each cookie.

7. Bake for 12 (for soft cookies) to 14 minutes (for crisper cookies) or until very lightly browned on the bottom. Remove from the oven. Let cool slightly before transferring cookies to a rack to cool completely. Store cookies in an airtight container at room temperature.

Variation: You can replace the natural peanut butter with freshly ground almond butter or other nut or seed butter as desired.

MEATLESS AND WHEATLESS

We recommend making these cookies with natural peanut butter made just from freshly ground roasted peanuts, which you can either purchase from a grind-your-own dispenser or make at home using a food processor. If you want to use a jarred peanut butter (or other nut or seed butter variety) instead, only add 2 tablespoons sunflower oil to the cookie batter. The jarred peanut butter has a different consistency due to the oil and other ingredients in it, so you don't need as much other oil.

Quinoa Flake Cookies with Cranberries, Raisins, and Walnuts

Slightly nutty *quinoa flakes* and flour, plus golden millet and sorghum flours, give these cookies a wholesomeness, which is perfect for the additions of crunchy walnuts, raisins, dried cranberries, and a sweet blend of maple syrup and date paste.

Yield:	Prep time:	Cook time:	Serving size:
2 dozen cookies	5 to 7 minutes	12 to 14 minutes	2 cookies

6 TB. water

¼ cup Date Paste (recipe in Chapter 8)

¼ cup maple syrup

3 TB. sunflower or other oil

1 tsp. alcohol-free vanilla extract

1½ cups quinoa flakes

1 cup millet flour

¾ cup sorghum flour

¾ cup quinoa flour

½ cup tapioca starch

1 tsp. ground cinnamon

1 tsp. baking soda

½ tsp. gluten-free xanthan gum

½ tsp. sea salt

¼ cup dried cranberries

¼ cup raisins

¼ cup raw walnuts, roughly chopped

1. Preheat the oven to 350°F. Line 2 large cookie sheets with parchment paper or Silpat liners.

2. In a food processor fitted with an S blade, place water, Date Paste, maple syrup, sunflower oil, and vanilla extract, and process for 1 minute. Scrape down the sides of the container with a spatula, and process for 30 more seconds.

3. In a medium bowl, combine quinoa flakes, millet flour, sorghum flour, quinoa flour, tapioca starch, cinnamon, baking soda, xanthan gum, and sea salt, and stir well to combine.

4. Add wet ingredients to dry ingredients, and stir well to combine. Stir in dried cranberries, raisins, and walnuts.

5. Portion cookie dough using a 2-inch scoop or heaping 2 tablespoonfuls onto the prepared cookie sheets, spacing them 2 inches apart. Using your wet fingers, flatten each cookie slightly.

6. Bake for 12 to 14 minutes or until lightly golden brown on the bottom and around the edges. Remove from the oven. Let cool slightly before transferring cookies to a rack to cool completely. Store cookies in an airtight container at room temperature.

Variation: You can replace the dried cranberries and raisins with other varieties of dried fruit, such as currants, cherries, goji berries, or chopped dates. You can also replace the walnuts with chopped almonds, pecans, or whole sunflower or pumpkin seeds.

> **DEFINITION**
>
> **Quinoa flakes** are made from quinoa that's been prewashed to remove the bitter and protective saponin coating and steamrolled into a quick-cooking flake. Enjoy quinoa flakes cooked in liquid for a hot cereal, or use them as a replacement for rolled oats in baked goods. Ancient Harvest quinoa flakes are available in most grocery and natural foods stores.

Chocolate-Chip Cookies

These multi-grain cookies are rich, gooey, and chewy.

Yield:	Prep time:	Cook time:	Serving size:
2½ to 3 dozen cookies	10 minutes, plus 1 hour chill time	12 to 14 minutes	2 cookies

3 TB. water

1 TB. ground golden flaxseeds or flaxseed meal

⅔ cup nonhydrogenated margarine

½ cup unbleached cane sugar

½ cup turbinado sugar or vegan light brown sugar

1 tsp. alcohol-free vanilla extract

1½ cups Bob's Red Mill Gluten-Free All-Purpose Baking Flour

½ cup millet flour or quinoa flour

1½ tsp. gluten-free xanthan gum

1 tsp. aluminum-free baking powder

¾ tsp. baking soda

½ tsp. sea salt

1 cup vegan gluten-free chocolate chips or carob chips

1. Preheat the oven to 350°F. Line 2 large cookie sheets with parchment paper or Silpat liners.

2. In a large bowl, combine water and flaxseeds, and let sit for 5 minutes.

3. Add margarine, unbleached cane sugar, turbinado sugar, and vanilla extract, and stir together until light and creamy.

4. Add Bob's Red Mill Gluten-Free All-Purpose Baking Flour, millet flour, xanthan gum, baking powder, baking soda, and sea salt, and stir well until mixture forms a soft dough. Gently stir in chocolate chips. Cover and chill dough for 1 hour or until firm.

5. Portion cookie dough using a 2-inch scoop or heaping 2 tablespoonfuls onto the prepared cookie sheets, spacing them 2 inches apart. Using your wet fingers, flatten each cookie slightly.

6. Bake for 12 to 14 minutes or until lightly golden brown on the bottom and around the edges. Remove from the oven. Let cool slightly before transferring cookies to a rack to cool completely. Store cookies in an airtight container at room temperature.

Variation: Feel free to add ¹⁄₂ cup roughly chopped nuts or seeds as desired, or replace the chocolate chips with an equal amount of raisins or other dried fruit. To make **Chocolate-Chip Bar Cookies,** place the cookie dough in a lightly oiled 8×10-inch baking pan (or silicone baking pan) and bake for 22 to 25 minutes or until a toothpick inserted in the center comes out clean.

AGAINST THE GRAIN

The most readily available vegan carob chips brand, SunSpire, contains barley as a sweetener and, therefore, is not gluten free. Barry Farm Foods (barryfarm.com) sells several gluten-free vegan carob chips, including unsweetened and sugar-sweetened varieties.

Fudgy Brownies

By using a combination of melted chocolate chips, puréed bananas, and our Prune Paste, we've achieved a moist and chocolaty brownie without adding in any oil or margarine, so you don't have to feel guilty if you can't stop at just eating one!

Yield:	Prep time:	Cook time:	Serving size:
1 (9×13-inch) pan or 12 pieces	10 minutes	35 to 40 minutes	1 piece

1¹⁄₂ cups Beverly's Baking Blend (recipe in Chapter 3) or Bob's Red Mill Gluten-Free All-Purpose Baking Flour

6 TB. cocoa powder

1 tsp. gluten-free xanthan gum

¹⁄₂ tsp. aluminum-free baking powder

¹⁄₂ tsp. sea salt

1 (12-oz.) pkg. vegan gluten-free chocolate chips

3 medium bananas, peeled and cut into 2-in. pieces

¹⁄₂ cup Prune Paste (variation in Chapter 8)

²⁄₃ cup maple syrup

2 tsp. alcohol-free vanilla extract

²⁄₃ cup raw walnuts or other nuts, roughly chopped

1. Preheat the oven to 350°F. Lightly oil a 9×13-inch baking pan, or use a silicone baking pan.

2. In a large bowl, whisk together Beverly's Baking Blend, cocoa powder, xanthan gum, baking powder, and sea salt.

3. In the top of a *double boiler*, place chocolate chips, and heat until thoroughly melted. Remove from heat, and set aside. (Alternatively, you can melt chocolate chips in a microwave-safe bowl in the microwave, heating for 30-second increments until chocolate chips just begin to melt and stirring until smooth.)

4. In a food processor fitted with an S blade, combine bananas, Prune Paste, maple syrup, and vanilla extract, and process for 1 minute. Scrape down the sides of the container with a spatula, and process for 1 more minute or until smooth.

5. Add banana mixture and melted chocolate chips to dry ingredients, and stir well to combine. Transfer brownie batter to the prepared pan. Sprinkle chopped walnuts over top, and using your hands, gently press them into brownie batter.

6. Bake for 35 to 40 minutes or until center is set. Allow to cool completely, at least 1 hour or more, before cutting into 12 pieces.

Variation: For **Frosted Brownies,** don't sprinkle brownies with chopped walnuts prior to baking. Instead, immediately after removing the brownies from the oven, sprinkle an additional $1/2$ cup vegan chocolate chips over the top. When they've melted, gently spread them with a knife to completely cover the top of the brownies. Sprinkle the chopped walnuts over the top, and allow frosting to set completely before cutting brownies into pieces.

DEFINITION

A **double boiler** (a.k.a. bain-marie) consists of a set of two saucepans (or a medium bowl and a saucepan), placed one on top of the other. The bottom saucepan contains several inches of water and is placed over low heat to simmer, while the top saucepan (or bowl) contains the item to be melted or gently heated. A double boiler is typically used to melt chocolate.

Crispy Rice Trail Mix Bars

One of our homemade energy bars—made with crispy brown rice cereal, crunchy nuts and seeds, and chewy dried fruits all enrobed in a blend of nut butter and brown rice syrup—can help sustain you, whether you're out on a hike or just in need of an on-the-go breakfast.

Yield:	Prep time:	Cook time:	Serving size:
1 (9×13-inch) pan or 12 pieces	5 to 7 minutes, plus 30 minutes chill time	2 or 3 minutes	1 piece

4 cups gluten-free crispy brown rice cereal

¼ cup raw sliced almonds

¼ cup raw pumpkin seeds

¼ cup raw sunflower seeds

¼ cup goji berries

¼ cup dried apricots, cut into thin strips

¼ cup dried cherries or cranberries

¼ cup raisins or currants

2 TB. raw hemp seeds

1 cup gluten-free brown rice syrup

1 cup nut butter (such as almond, cashew, peanut, or sunflower butter)

½ tsp. ground cinnamon

¼ tsp. sea salt

1 TB. alcohol-free vanilla extract

1. Lightly oil a 9×13-inch baking pan, or use a silicone baking pan.

2. In a large bowl, combine crispy brown rice cereal, almonds, pumpkin seeds, sunflower seeds, goji berries, dried apricots, dried cherries, raisins, and hemp seeds.

3. In a medium saucepan, combine brown rice syrup, nut butter, cinnamon, and sea salt, and cook over low heat, stirring often, for 2 or 3 minutes or until creamy and small bubbles begin to appear. Remove from heat, and stir in vanilla extract.

4. Pour brown rice mixture over cereal mixture, and stir well until evenly coated. Transfer mixture to the prepared pan. Dampen your hands with water, and press mixture firmly into the pan.

5. Place pan in the refrigerator to chill for 30 minutes or until firm. Remove from the refrigerator and cut into 12 pieces. Store bars in an airtight container at room temperature.

Variation: Feel free to replace the nuts, seeds, and dried fruits with 1¾ to 2 cups your favorite packaged trail mix blend. For added fiber, replace ½ cup crispy rice cereal with ⅔ cup quinoa flakes and 2 tablespoons chia seeds.

AGAINST THE GRAIN

Be careful when stirring the brown rice syrup and nut butter mixture while it's heating because the smallest splash of the hot mixture can burn you. Also, when adding the vanilla extract, do so carefully because it will bubble up when it comes into contact with the hot mixture.

Nostalgic Sweet Treats

In This Chapter

- Mouth-watering mousse and pudding
- Luscious layered and filled treats
- Flavorful pie, crisp, and tarts

The desire to re-create some of our favorite childhood (and adulthood) desserts using gluten-free and vegan ingredients was the inspiration for this chapter. In it, you'll learn how easy it can be to change up a few ingredients here and there to reinvent some beloved comfort foods, as well as a few café-style creations, so you can once again enjoy sweet treats to your heart and tummy's content.

Fruits, nuts, and nondairy milks feature predominantly in many of these recipes. You learn how to easily blend or cook them into tasty treats, like Sweet Nut Crème, Berry Tofu Mousse, and Tapioca Pudding, as well as to artistically layer your components to make Raw Fruit Parfaits. We also show you how to make your own veganized cream puffs using baked mochi and a Vegan Pastry Cream.

We also share recipes for making a baked fruit crisp, two types of tarts, and your very own gluten-free vegan pie. So head to your kitchen and get ready to create some sweet treats!

Plant-Based Dietitian Recommends: Sweet Nut Crème, Berry Tofu Mousse, Tapioca Pudding, and Raw Fruit Parfaits are excellent, nutritious dessert options. If you're trying to lose weight, focus on fresh fruit as staples and the others as special treats.

Sweet Nut Crème

This light and creamy topping is made with a mixture of raw cashews, dried dates, coconut water, and vanilla extract. It can be used in place of a tofu-based whipped topping on your favorite desserts.

Yield:	Prep time:	Serving size:
1½ cups	5 minutes, plus 6 hours or more soak time	2 or 3 tablespoons

1½ cups water
1½ cups raw cashews
6 dried dates, pitted

⅓ cup unsweetened coconut water (or additional water)
1 tsp. alcohol-free vanilla extract or ½ tsp. raw vanilla bean powder

1. In a medium bowl, combine water, cashews, and dates, and set aside to soak for 6 hours or overnight.

2. Drain off soaking water, rinse cashews and dates, and drain again.

3. Transfer cashews and dates to a food processor fitted with an S blade. Add coconut water and vanilla extract, and process for 1 minute. Scrape down the sides of the container with a spatula, and process for 1 more minute or until light and creamy.

4. Transfer nut crème to an airtight container, and store in the refrigerator for up to 1 week. Use as a topping for puddings, pies, or your other favorite desserts or sweet treats.

Variation: You can also make this sweet nut crème with a mixture of raw nuts, such as macadamias, pine nuts, and cashews. For **Almond Nut Crème,** soak only 4 dried dates in some water for 30 minutes or until soft, and drain and discard the soaking liquid. Replace the cashews with 1 cup almond meal pulp from making Awesome Almond Milk (recipe in Chapter 4), use 3 tablespoons coconut water and ¾ teaspoon vanilla extract, and process ingredients in similar manner as directed.

CORNUCOPIA

We suggest soaking raw nuts and seeds in many of our recipes because all raw nuts and seeds contain growth inhibitors that help keep them from sprouting prematurely if they happen to get wet. This is all part of nature's way of protecting them so they'll only grow under optimal conditions. Plus, the soaking makes the raw nuts and seeds more easily digestible.

Berry Tofu Mousse

When blended, silken tofu becomes ultra creamy, and with the addition of some binders, berries, sugar, and vanilla extract, unassuming tofu is magically metamorphosized into a flavorful dairy-free *mousse*.

Yield:	Prep time:	Cook time:	Serving size:
3 cups	5 to 7 minutes, plus 1 hour chill time	3 or 4 minutes	⅔ cup

2½ cups fresh strawberries, blueberries, or raspberries, or a mixture or 1 (16-oz.) pkg. frozen berries of choice (thawed)

1 (12-oz.) pkg. firm or extra-firm silken tofu

⅓ cup unbleached cane sugar or gluten-free brown rice syrup

1 tsp. alcohol-free vanilla extract

2 TB. plus ¾ cup water or unsweetened coconut water

2 TB. cornstarch or arrowroot

2 tsp. agar powder

1. In a blender or food processor fitted with an S blade, combine berries, silken tofu, unbleached cane sugar, and vanilla extract, and process for 1 minute. Scrape down the sides of the container with a spatula, and process for 30 more seconds.

2. In a small bowl, combine 2 tablespoons water and cornstarch, and set aside.

3. In a small saucepan, combine remaining ¾ cup water and agar powder, and cook over medium heat, stirring often, for 2 minutes. Stir in cornstarch mixture, and cook, stirring often, for 1 more minute or until it becomes a thickened, gel-like mixture. Remove from heat.

4. Add agar mixture to food processor, and process for 1 minute. Scrape down the sides of the container with a spatula, and process for 30 more seconds.

5. Transfer berry mousse to an airtight container and chill for 1 hour or more. Serve cold or at room temperature, plain, or top individual servings with a dollop of Sweet Nut Crème (recipe earlier in this chapter), and/or a few additional fresh berries or sliced fruit as desired.

Variation: You can make other fruit-flavored tofu mousse by replacing the berries with an equal amount of your favorite fruit, such as peaches, mangoes, or bananas.

DEFINITION

Mousse in French translates as "lather" or "foam." Most people associate the term with a light and creamy puddinglike dessert. In classic French cooking, a mousse is often prepared with a mixture of heavy cream, beaten eggs (or egg whites), dissolved gelatin, sugar, and melted chocolate, fruit purées, or other flavoring ingredients.

Tapioca Pudding

Tapioca pudding, like rice pudding, is a comfort food many of us grew up with. This slightly sweet, ultra-creamy pudding is easy to prepare using our Sweetened Vanilla Almond Milk, small *tapioca pearls*, brown rice syrup, and vanilla extract.

Yield:	Prep time:	Cook time:	Serving size:
2½ to 3 cups	5 minutes, plus 1 hour soak time	22 to 25 minutes	⅔ cup

2 TB. plus 2 cups unsweetened coconut water or water

1 TB. arrowroot or cornstarch

⅓ cup small tapioca pearls

2 cups Sweet Vanilla Almond Milk (variation in Chapter 4) or vanilla-flavored soy milk or other nondairy milk

¼ cup gluten-free brown rice syrup

¼ tsp. sea salt

1½ tsp. alcohol-free vanilla extract or ¾ tsp. raw vanilla bean powder

1. In a small bowl, combine 2 tablespoons coconut water and arrowroot, and set aside.

2. In a large saucepan, combine remaining 2 cups coconut water and tapioca pearls, and set aside to soak for 1 hour.

3. Stir Sweet Vanilla Almond Milk, brown rice syrup, and sea salt into tapioca mixture, and bring to a boil over high heat. Reduce heat to low, and cook, stirring constantly to prevent scorching, for 20 minutes or until tapioca pearls soften a bit and become transparent.

4. Stir in arrowroot mixture, and cook, stirring constantly, for 2 or 3 more minutes or until thickened. Remove from heat, and stir in vanilla extract.

5. Transfer tapioca pudding to a large bowl or individual serving bowls as desired. Serve warm or cold, plain, or topped with a dollop of Sweet Nut Crème (recipe earlier in this chapter) as desired. Store tapioca pudding covered in the refrigerator.

Variation: For **Chocolate Tapioca Pudding,** replace the Sweet Vanilla Almond Milk with an equal amount of chocolate-flavored soy or almond milk.

> **DEFINITION**
>
> **Tapioca pearls** are made from tapioca starch (a.k.a. tapioca flour), which is derived from the cassava plant. The tapioca starch is soaked, cooked, shaped, and dried into assorted-size pellets (or pearls, as they're commonly referred to). White, small tapioca pearls, as well as granulated (quick-cooking) tapioca, are available packaged in most grocery stores.

Raw Fruit Parfaits

These beautiful parfaits resemble an old-fashioned ice cream sundae in appearance but are a healthier option. They're made by alternating layers of mixed fresh fruit, a date and orange–sweetened peach purée, shredded coconut, and sliced almonds.

Yield:	Prep time:	Serving size:
7 cups or 4 parfaits	10 to 15 minutes, plus 20 minutes soak time	1¾ cups or 1 parfait

⅔ cup dried dates, pitted

⅔ cup orange juice

1½ lb. (about 3 or 4 cups) fresh or frozen peaches, sliced (thawed)

¾ cup blueberries

¾ cup red raspberries or blackberries, cut in half lengthwise

¾ cup strawberries, hulled and sliced

1 large mango, peeled, pitted, and diced

1 kiwi, peeled, cut into quarters lengthwise, and thinly sliced

8 tsp. unsweetened shredded coconut or ¼ cup unsweetened coconut chips

¼ cup raw sliced almonds

1. In a small bowl, combine dates and orange juice, and set aside for 20 minutes to soften dates.

2. In a blender, place date mixture and peaches, and blend for 1 or 2 minutes or until smooth. Scrape down the sides of the container with a spatula, and blend for 1 more minute or until a very light and creamy purée.

3. In a medium bowl, combine blueberries, red raspberries, strawberries, mango, and kiwi.

4. To assemble parfaits: in the bottom of 4 large glasses or dessert dishes, layer, in order, ⅓ cup peach purée, ½ cup mixed fruit mixture, 1 teaspoon shredded coconut, and ½ tablespoon sliced almonds. Repeat layers. Serve immediately or chill for 30 minutes or more.

Variation: For a **Raw Fruit Trifle,** assemble components in a large glass bowl, placing half of peach purée, half of mixed fruit mixture, half of shredded coconut, and half of sliced almonds. Repeat layers.

CORNUCOPIA

When you talk about pectin, most cooks think of the packaged gelling agent used to thicken jellies and jams. Actually, pectin is a natural dietary fiber found in berries, apples, and other fruits, as well as some vegetables. Soaking, mashing, or cooking certain fruits and vegetables causes them to release their natural pectin, which will bind or thicken your dish—a process that can be very beneficial to gluten-free vegan cooking and baking.

Mochi Cream Puffs with Vegan Pastry Cream

Traditionally, cream puffs are made with *pâté à choux*, which is a cooked combination of flour, butter, and eggs. But thanks to Grainaissance *mochi*, gluten-free vegans can create a similar-style stuffed sweet treat.

Yield:	Prep time:		Cook time:	Serving size:
18 pieces	15 to 20 minutes, plus 30 minutes chill time		15 to 20 minutes	3 pieces

2 cups soy creamer or other non-dairy milk	1 tsp. alcohol-free vanilla extract or ¹⁄₂ tsp. raw vanilla bean powder
¹⁄₄ cup unbleached cane sugar or gluten-free brown rice syrup	2 (12.5-oz.) pkg. Grainaissance mochi (flavor of choice)
¹⁄₄ cup cornstarch	

1. In a small saucepan, whisk together soy creamer, unbleached cane sugar, and cornstarch, and cook over medium heat, whisking often, for 5 to 7 minutes or until thickened. Remove from heat, and whisk in vanilla extract. Pour **Vegan Pastry Cream** into a glass bowl, cover with parchment paper or plastic wrap, and chill for 30 minutes.

2. Preheat the oven to 450°F. Line a cookie sheet with parchment paper or a Silpat liner.

3. Meanwhile, using a sharp knife, cut each package of mochi into 9 square pieces (each about 1¹⁄₂×2 inches), for a total of 18 pieces. Place mochi pieces on the prepared cookie sheet, spacing them at least 1 inch apart.

4. Bake for 8 to 10 minutes or until mochi pieces puff up and are lightly browned around the edges. Remove from the oven, and let cool for 5 minutes. Using the tip of a knife, cut a slit along one side of each mochi piece, and allow mochi pieces to cool completely.

5. Using a spoon or a pastry bag, fill each mochi piece with $1\frac{1}{2}$ to 2 tablespoons chilled Vegan Pastry Cream. Serve immediately. If not serving all mochi pieces at one time, only fill mochi pieces with Vegan Pastry Cream as needed.

Variation: For a **Chocolate Vegan Pastry Cream,** whisk $\frac{1}{4}$ cup cocoa powder or raw cacao powder into the other Vegan Pastry Cream ingredients prior to heating. You can also fill your mochi puffs with an equal amount of chilled Berry Tofu Mousse (recipe earlier in this chapter).

DEFINITION

Mochi (pronounced *mo-chee*) is made from sweet short-grain brown rice that's been steamed and pounded, mashed, or finely ground and allowed to cool before being shaped into blocks. Mochi has a slightly chewy texture when baked and can be enjoyed as a snack or used for preparing sweet or savory recipes. It's available in assorted flavors in the refrigerated case of most grocery and natural foods stores.

Fall Fruit Crisp

Sliced apples and pears are lightly spiced and sweetened with apple juice and turbinado sugar to make a tasty filling. Many of these same components are combined with quinoa flakes and flour to create the crispy topping for this oven-baked dessert.

Yield:	Prep time:	Cook time:	Serving size:
1 (9-inch) pan or 4 servings	7 to 10 minutes	30 minutes	1 cup

2 large Gala apples or other apples, cored and thinly sliced

2 large Anjou, Bartlett, or Bosc pears, cored and thinly sliced

$\frac{1}{4}$ cup plus $\frac{1}{3}$ cup apple juice or water

$\frac{1}{2}$ cup turbinado sugar

2 TB. plus $\frac{1}{3}$ cup quinoa flour or other gluten-free flour of choice

1 tsp. alcohol-free vanilla extract

$1\frac{1}{2}$ tsp. ground cinnamon

$\frac{1}{2}$ tsp. ground ginger or ground cardamom

1 cup quinoa flakes

$\frac{1}{4}$ cup nonhydrogenated margarine or sunflower oil

1. Preheat the oven to 375°F.

2. In a medium bowl, combine apples, pears, $\frac{1}{4}$ cup apple juice, $\frac{1}{4}$ cup turbinado sugar, 2 tablespoons quinoa flour, vanilla extract, 1 teaspoon cinnamon, and ginger, and stir well. Transfer mixture to a 9-inch baking pan, or use a silicone baking pan.

3. In a small bowl, combine quinoa flakes, remaining $\frac{1}{4}$ cup turbinado sugar, remaining $\frac{1}{3}$ cup quinoa flour, and remaining $\frac{1}{2}$ teaspoon cinnamon. Using your fingers, work remaining $\frac{1}{3}$ cup apple juice and margarine into dry ingredients until mixture resembles coarse crumbs.

4. Sprinkle topping mixture over fruit filling. Bake for 30 minutes or until filling is bubbly and topping is lightly browned. Remove from the oven.

5. Serve warm or at room temperature, plain, or top individual servings with a dollop of Sweet Nut Crème (recipe earlier in this chapter) or scoops of nondairy ice cream or sorbet as desired.

Variation: For added crunch, to the topping mixture, add ¼ cup roughly chopped walnuts (or other nuts) or 2 tablespoons sunflower seeds or hemp seeds.

MEATLESS AND WHEATLESS

The easiest way to add variety to your daily diet is to adopt a seasonal approach to buying produce. When they're harvested during the appropriate season and not rushed to market, fresh produce items really are at their most flavorful and textural best. This is especially true for fresh fruit. So use this fruit crisp recipe simply as a starting-off point, and replace the apples and pears with rhubarb, berries, peaches, plums, or other seasonal fruits.

Favorite Fruit Pie

You call all the shots with this double-crusted, fruit-filled pie. We provide the know-how but leave the fruit selection, sweetening, and filling spicing all up to you.

Yield:	Prep time:	Cook time:	Serving size:
1 (9-inch) pie or 8 pieces	20 minutes, plus 30 minutes chill time	40 to 45 minutes	1 piece

5 cups whole fruit or berries or 6 cups thinly sliced fruit

⅔ cup plus 1 TB. turbinado sugar or unbleached cane sugar

¼ cup tapioca starch

2 tsp. lemon juice

1 tsp. ground cinnamon

½ tsp. additional spice of choice or a combination of spices (such as ground ginger, ground cardamom, freshly grated nutmeg, etc.)

¼ tsp. sea salt

1 batch pastry for Double Gluten-Free Piecrust (variation in Chapter 5) or double batch Single Sweetened Gluten-Free Piecrust (variation in Chapter 5)

1 TB. nondairy milk of choice

1. Preheat the oven to 350°F.

2. In a large bowl, combine fruit, ⅔ cup turbinado sugar, tapioca starch, lemon juice, cinnamon, additional spice(s), and sea salt, and set aside.

3. Prepare pastry for Double Gluten-Free Piecrust according to recipe instructions and chill 2 pastry dough discs for 30 minutes.

4. For easier rolling, place each chilled pastry dough disc between 2 (12×16-inch) pieces of parchment paper, and roll each into a 12-inch circle.

5. Work with one rolled-out pastry dough at a time, and set the other aside. Remove and discard top sheet of parchment paper. Flip pastry dough into a pie pan, and remove and discard remaining parchment paper.

6. Spoon pie filling mixture into bottom piecrust. Remove and discard top sheet of parchment paper from remaining rolled-out pastry dough. Flip pastry dough over top of pie filling, and remove and discard remaining parchment paper. Trim overhanging edge of both crusts about 1 inch from the outer edge of the pie pan. Gently press down on outer edges to seal and *flute* edges as desired.

7. Using a knife, cut 3 slits into top crust. Brush top crust with nondairy milk, and sprinkle remaining 1 tablespoon turbinado sugar over top.

8. Bake for 40 to 45 minutes or until crust is lightly browned. Remove from the oven. Allow pie to cool for at least 1 hour before cutting.

9. Serve warm or room temperature, plain, or top individual servings with a dollop of Sweet Nut Crème (recipe earlier in this chapter) or scoops of nondairy ice cream or sorbet as desired.

Variation: For a maple-sweetened pie, replace the turbinado sugar in the filling with $\frac{1}{3}$ cup maple syrup, and instead of brushing nondairy milk on the top crust, use 1 tablespoon maple syrup instead. To make a **Free-Form Fruit Pie** (a.k.a. a galette), make a Single Sweetened Gluten-Free Piecrust (variation in Chapter 5), chill for 30 minutes, and roll pastry dough into a 14-inch circle between sheets of parchment paper. Transfer to a large cookie sheet, and remove and discard top sheet of parchment paper. Mound pie filling in the center of the circle, fold up edges of the pastry dough to make a 3-inch-wide border around the filling, crimping and pleating as needed to maintain a circular pattern. Bake for 25 to 30 minutes.

DEFINITION

In most pie recipes, you're instructed to **flute** the edges, giving your piecrust a decorative border edge. The simplest fluted finish is done by pressing the tines of a fork into the pastry dough, going all the way around the outer edge. For a fancier fluted edge, push the outer edge of pastry dough in with the thumb and index finger of one hand, while pressing or pinching toward it with the index finger of your other hand.

Berries and Cream Tart

We've placed our Gluten-Free Piecrust in a *tart pan* as the base for this fruit tart, which is filled with our silky, smooth Vegan Pastry Cream and decoratively topped with an assortment of fresh berries.

Yield:	Prep time:	Cook time:	Serving size:
1 (9-inch) tart or 8 pieces	15 to 20 minutes, plus 30 to 40 minutes chill time	10 to 15 minutes	1 piece

1 batch pastry for Gluten-Free Piecrust (recipe in Chapter 5) or Single Sweetened Gluten-Free Piecrust (variation in Chapter 5)

1 batch Vegan Pastry Cream (recipe earlier in this chapter), chilled

1½ cups fresh strawberries, hulled and sliced

1 cup fresh blueberries

1 cup fresh red raspberries or blackberries

1. Preheat the oven to 350°F. Lightly oil a 9-inch tart pan with a removable bottom, or use a nonstick tart pan.

2. Prepare pastry for Gluten-Free Piecrust according to recipe instructions, and chill dough disc for 30 minutes.

3. For easier rolling, place chilled pastry dough disc between 2 (12×16-inch) pieces of parchment paper, and roll into a 12-inch circle. Remove and discard top sheet of parchment paper.

4. Flip pastry dough into tart pan, and remove and discard remaining parchment paper. Using your hands, firmly press pastry dough to cover the bottom and sides of the prepared tart pan.

5. Place tart pan on a large cookie sheet, and bake for 10 to 15 minutes or until lightly browned and set. Remove from the oven. Allow tart crust to cool completely.

6. Remove outer ring from tart pan, and place cooled tart crust on a large plate or platter.

7. Spoon chilled Vegan Pastry Cream into tart crust. Decoratively arrange sliced strawberries, blueberries, and red raspberries over top as desired. Cut tart into 8 pieces and serve immediately, or chill for 30 minutes and cut it into pieces.

Variation: For a **Very Berry Tart,** replace the Vegan Pastry Cream with Berry Tofu Mousse (recipe earlier in this chapter), and top the mousse with fresh berries as described. To adapt this recipe to make a really stunning **Fresh Fruit Tart,** decorate the top of the tart instead using only ¾ cup sliced strawberries and ½ cup each blueberries and raspberries, and combine them with 2 cups whole or sliced assorted fresh fruits, such as peaches, nectarines, kiwi, mango, banana, or grapes.

DEFINITION

Tart pans have either fluted or straight sides, in contrast to pie pans, which are sloped. Many tart pans feature a removable bottom and outer ring construction, which makes transferring the finished tart or quiche to a plate or cake stand for serving easy. They're available in a variety of sizes and shapes, including round, square, and rectangular, as well as in both metal and nonstick finishes.

Mixed Nut Tart

You'll go nuts over this tart! It features ground nuts in the crust plus a filling made with a generous combination of shelled nuts, almond milk, spices, and sweet brown rice and maple syrups.

Yield:	Prep time:	Cook time:	Serving size:
1 (9-inch) tart or 8 pieces	15 to 20 minutes	35 to 40 minutes	1 piece

$\frac{1}{3}$ cup raw pecan pieces or whole pecans

$\frac{1}{3}$ cup demerara sugar or turbinado sugar

1 cup brown rice flour

$\frac{1}{3}$ cup plus 1 TB. arrowroot

$\frac{1}{4}$ cup tapioca starch

$\frac{1}{2}$ tsp. gluten-free xanthan gum

$\frac{1}{3}$ cup nonhydrogenated margarine

3 TB. water

$2\frac{1}{2}$ cups mixed raw nuts (such as a combination of almonds, hazelnuts, pecans, and/or walnuts)

$\frac{2}{3}$ cup gluten-free brown rice syrup

$\frac{2}{3}$ cup maple syrup

1 tsp. ground cinnamon

1 tsp. ground ginger

$\frac{1}{2}$ tsp. freshly grated nutmeg

$\frac{1}{4}$ tsp. sea salt

$\frac{1}{4}$ cup flaxseeds or golden flaxseeds

$\frac{1}{2}$ cup Awesome Almond Milk (recipe in Chapter 4) or other nondairy milk

1 TB. alcohol-free vanilla extract

1. Preheat the oven to 375°F. Lightly oil a 9-inch tart pan with a removable bottom, or use a nonstick tart pan.

2. In a food processor fitted with an S blade, place pecans and demerara sugar, and process for 1 minute or until pecans are finely chopped. Add brown rice flour, $\frac{1}{3}$ cup arrowroot, tapioca starch, and xanthan gum, and process for 30 seconds.

3. Add margarine and process for 1 minute or until mixture resembles coarse crumbs. Scrape down the sides of the container with a spatula. While the machine is running, through the feed tube, slowly drizzle in water, and process for 30 to 60 seconds or until mixture just starts to come together into a ball.

4. Transfer crust mixture to the prepared tart pan. Using your hands, firmly press mixture to evenly cover the bottom and sides of the tart pan. Place the tart pan on a large cookie sheet, and bake for 5 minutes. Remove from the oven.

5. Place mixed nuts into tart crust, and bake for 5 to 7 more minutes or until nuts are lightly toasted and fragrant. Remove from the oven.

6. Meanwhile, in a small saucepan, combine brown rice syrup, maple syrup, cinnamon, ginger, nutmeg, and sea salt. Bring to a boil over high heat, reduce heat to low, and simmer for 5 minutes. Remove from heat.

7. In a blender, place flaxseeds, and blend for 1 or 2 minutes or until finely ground. Add Awesome Almond Milk and remaining 1 tablespoon arrowroot, and process for 30 seconds.

8. Add warm brown rice syrup mixture and vanilla extract, and process for 30 more seconds. Scrape down the sides of the container with a spatula, and process for 30 more seconds.

9. Pour brown rice syrup mixture over toasted nuts in tart crust, and bake for 30 to 35 more minutes or until filling is bubbling. Remove from the oven. Allow tart to cool on cookie sheet for 5 minutes, and transfer to a rack to cool completely.

10. Remove outer ring from the tart pan, and place tart on a large plate or platter. Cut into 8 pieces, and serve plain, or top individual servings with a dollop of Sweet Nut Crème (recipe earlier in this chapter) or scoops of nondairy ice cream or sorbet as desired. Cover extra tart with plastic wrap, and store in the refrigerator.

Variation: In the tart crust, you can replace the pecans with an equal amount of other nuts or almond meal. To adapt this recipe to make a **Mixed Nut and Seed Tart,** use a combination of $1\frac{1}{2}$ cups raw mixed nuts and 1 cup raw mixed seeds (such as sunflower seeds, pumpkin seeds, and hemp seeds) in filling mixture. For a **Pecan Pie,** use a Single Sweetened Gluten-Free Piecrust (variation in Chapter 5), and replace the mixed nuts in the filling mixture with 3 cups whole pecans or pecan pieces. Assemble and bake pie as directed.

MEATLESS AND WHEATLESS

During the holidays, it's nearly impossible to find gluten-free vegan pies at your local grocery store. But now you don't have to go without! Just bake one yourself! This recipe and the variations are all perfect for serving on special occasions.

Occasional Indulgences

In This Chapter

- Glazing, saucing, and frosting your desserts
- Bountiful baked cakes
- Silky tofu-based no-bake cake and cheesecake

In this chapter, we provide several over-the-top dessert recipes, all of which are sweetened in one way or another. In some of the more involved recipes, we've used several different types of sweeteners. That's why we titled this chapter "Occasional Indulgences." We encourage you to eat healthfully as part of your daily routine. If you do, you can allow yourself an occasional luxury or sweet treat.

Have we piqued your curiosity about what lies ahead? Well then, let's get to it! We start off with two tasty toppings—After Dark Glaze and Caramel Rum Sauce. We then move on to cakes—cakes of every shape and size, like Lemon-Yogurt Pound Cake, petite-size Mini Chocolate Bundt Cakes, and oil-free and citrus-sweetened Pecan Carrot Cake. We finish the chapter with some deliciously decadent silken tofu-based creations, including a no-bake Chocolate Mousse Cake with Quinoa Crust and a lusciously simple Vegan Cheesecake.

Turn the page to see how delicious gluten-free vegan desserts can be!

After Dark Glaze

This ultra-rich, chocolaty glaze gets its deep, dark flavor from a combination of coffee, cocoa powder, and a chopped dark chocolate bar. It's so good you'll be tempted to eat it by the spoonful!

Yield:	Prep time:	Cook time:	Serving size:
1½ cups	2 minutes, plus 5 minutes cool time	3 minutes	3 tablespoons

¾ cup maple syrup

1 (3-oz.) vegan gluten-free dark chocolate bar, roughly chopped, or 1 cup vegan gluten-free chocolate chips

6 TB. cocoa powder or *raw cacao powder*

6 TB. hot or cold coffee or decaf coffee

⅛ tsp. sea salt

1 TB. alcohol-free vanilla extract

1. In a small saucepan, combine maple syrup, chopped chocolate bar, cocoa powder, coffee, and sea salt, and cook over medium heat, whisking often, for 3 minutes. Remove from heat. Whisk in vanilla extract.

2. Allow glaze to cool for 5 minutes to thicken slightly. Use as a topping for cakes, nondairy ice cream or sorbet, or on your other favorite desserts as desired. Store glaze in an airtight container in the refrigerator.

Variation: If you don't have any coffee on hand, use an equal amount of water instead. For a spiced glaze, add ¼ teaspoon ground cinnamon or cayenne.

DEFINITION

Raw cacao powder is made from raw cacao beans that have gone through a cold-pressing process to remove the fat (cacao butter) and then are finely ground into a powder, much like cocoa powder (which is made from roasted cacao beans). It has a deep, dark, almost coffeelike flavor; is rich in antioxidants; and is often used by raw foodists and others as a replacement for cocoa powder in recipes.

Caramel Rum Sauce

Cooking down soy creamer with some brown rice and maple syrups drastically shortens the time it takes to make caramel sauce. And to give this luscious sauce a little extra something in the flavor department, we've added a generous shot of rum.

Yield:	Prep time:	Cook time:	Serving size:
1½ cups	2 minutes	5 to 7 minutes	2 or 3 tablespoons

1 cup plain or vanilla soy creamer or nondairy milk of choice

6 TB. gluten-free brown rice syrup

6 TB. maple syrup

2 TB. cold water

2 TB. arrowroot

3 TB. light or dark rum

2 tsp. alcohol-free vanilla extract

1. In a small saucepan, combine soy creamer, brown rice syrup, and maple syrup, and cook over medium heat, whisking often, for 3 minutes.

2. In a small bowl, combine cold water and arrowroot. Add arrowroot mixture to the saucepan, and cook, whisking often, for 2 or 3 more minutes or until thickened. Remove from heat, and whisk in rum and vanilla extract.

3. Serve warm, at room temperature, or chilled as desired. Use as a topping for pies, fruit crisp, cakes, nondairy ice cream or sorbet, or your other favorite desserts as desired. Store sauce in an airtight container in the refrigerator.

Variation: For an alcohol-free caramel sauce, omit rum, and add an additional 1 tablespoon vanilla extract instead.

MEATLESS AND WHEATLESS

If you're fond of caramel apples, dip apple slices or a whole apple on a stick into warm or chilled Caramel Rum Sauce. If you're sharing with a little one (a.k.a. under-age person), make the alcohol-free variation.

Banana Bread Pudding with Caramel Rum Sauce

We love to use a loaf of our freshly baked Banana-Date Bread, soaked in a sweetened soy-based custard, layered with sliced bananas and chopped nuts, in this banana bread pudding.

Yield:	Prep time:	Cook time:	Serving size:
1 (8×10-inch) pan or 6 servings	10 to 15 minutes, plus 30 minutes soak time	40 to 45 minutes	1½ cups

1 loaf Banana-Date Bread (recipe in Chapter 5)

2 cups plain or vanilla soy creamer, or other nondairy milk

½ cup maple syrup or gluten-free brown rice syrup

2 tsp. cornstarch or tapioca starch

½ tsp. ground cinnamon

2 tsp. alcohol-free vanilla extract

2 medium bananas, peeled and sliced

½ cup raw walnuts, roughly chopped

2 TB. *demerara sugar* or *turbinado sugar*

1 batch Carmel Rum Sauce (recipe earlier in this chapter)

1. Cut Banana-Date Bread into ½-inch-thick slices, and cut slices into ½-inch cubes. Place bread cubes in a large bowl, and set aside.

2. In a small saucepan, whisk together soy creamer, maple syrup, cornstarch, and cinnamon, and bring to a boil over high heat. Reduce heat to low, and cook, whisking often, for 1 more minute. Remove from heat, and whisk in vanilla extract.

3. Pour soy creamer mixture over bread cubes, stir gently to combine, and set aside to soak for 30 minutes.

4. Preheat the oven to 375°F. Lightly oil a 8×10-inch baking pan, or use a silicone baking pan.

5. To assemble bread pudding, layer, in order, half of bread cube mixture, 1 sliced banana, and ¼ cup chopped walnuts. Repeat layers. Evenly sprinkle demerara sugar over top.

6. Bake for 40 to 45 minutes or until sugar is caramelized and top is golden brown and slightly crisp. Remove from the oven.

7. Serve warm, and over individual servings, drizzle a little Caramel Rum Sauce. Cover extra bread pudding with plastic wrap, and store in the refrigerator.

Variation: For an over-the-top banana-flavored treat, serve scoops of nondairy ice cream on top of each individual serving, with Caramel Rum Sauce drizzled over top. You can also add ¼ cup vegan gluten-free chocolate chips when assembling the layers. For **Chocolate Lover's Bread Pudding,** replace the Banana-Date Bread with cubes of Chocolate, Chocolate Chip, and Raspberry Bread (recipe in Chapter 5), replace the soy creamer with chocolate nondairy milk, assemble and bake as directed, and top individual servings with a drizzle of After Dark Glaze (recipe earlier in this chapter).

DEFINITION

Demerara sugar is a large, coarsely granulated variety of cane sugar that hails from the Demerara region of Guyana. It has a golden amber color and slight molasses flavor and can be used as a replacement for light or dark brown sugar in recipes. Bakers use demerara sugar to give a sweet, crunchy topping to muffins and other baked goods. **Turbinado sugar** is made from the juice extracted from unrefined raw cane sugar, which is then spun in a centrifuge or turbine. It has a very fine texture, a slight molasses flavor, and can be used to replace light brown sugar.

Lemon-Yogurt Pound Cake

This pound cake is moist and dense with a delightful lemony flavor.

Yield:	Prep time:	Cook time:	Serving size:
1 (8×4×2½-inch) pound cake	8 to 10 minutes	35 to 40 minutes	1 slice

1½ cups Bob's Red Mill Gluten-Free All-Purpose Baking Flour

⅔ cup unbleached cane sugar

¼ cup millet flour

¾ tsp. aluminum-free baking powder

¾ tsp. baking soda

½ tsp. gluten-free xanthan gum

¼ tsp. sea salt

2 TB. cold water

1 TB. Ener-G Egg Replacer

½ cup vanilla or lemon vegan yogurt

Zest of 1 large lemon

Juice of 1 large lemon

3 TB. sunflower oil or other oil

1 tsp. alcohol-free vanilla extract

½ cup seltzer water

1. Preheat the oven to 375°F. Lightly oil a 8×4×2½-inch loaf pan, or use a silicone loaf pan.

2. In a large bowl, combine Bob's Red Mill Gluten-Free All-Purpose Baking Flour, unbleached cane sugar, millet flour, baking powder, baking soda, xanthan gum, and sea salt, and whisk well to combine.

3. In a medium bowl, combine cold water and Ener-G Egg Replacer, and whisk vigorously for 1 minute or until very frothy (like beaten egg whites).

4. Add vanilla yogurt, lemon zest, lemon juice, sunflower oil, and vanilla extract, and whisk well to combine.

5. Add yogurt mixture and seltzer water to dry ingredients, and whisk well to combine.

6. Transfer batter to the prepared pan, and bake for 35 to 40 minutes or until a toothpick inserted in the center comes out clean. Remove from the oven. Allow loaf to cool slightly in the pan, and transfer to a rack to cool as desired.

7. Serve warm or at room temperature, plain, glazed, or frosted as desired. Store pound cake in an airtight container or cover with plastic wrap and store at room temperature.

Variation: For a **Lemon Poppy Seed Pound Cake,** stir 1½ tablespoons poppy seeds into the batter prior to baking. You can also make this recipe using limes, oranges, blood oranges, satsumas, or tangerines, using ¼ cup citrus juice and 1 tablespoon zest.

MEATLESS AND WHEATLESS

Often for an added touch, pound cakes are topped with glaze or frosting. For lemon glaze, stir together ½ cup unbleached sugar and 1 tablespoon lemon juice in a small saucepan, cook over low heat until sugar is dissolved, and pour over the pound cake. For lemony frosting, whisk together ½ cup vegan confectioners' sugar and 3 or 4 teaspoons lemon juice in a small bowl, adding lemon juice 1 teaspoon at a time, until mixture is smooth and thin enough to drizzle over the pound cake.

Vanilla Cupcakes with Buttercream Frosting

Our gluten-free vanilla cupcakes bake up light and moist. Topped with a flourish of vegan buttercream frosting, they're irresistible!

Yield:	Prep time:	Cook time:	Serving size:
12 cupcakes	15 to 20 minutes, plus 30 minutes cool time	20 to 22 minutes	1 cupcake

2¼ cups Beverly's Baking Blend (recipe in Chapter 3)

¾ cup unbleached cane sugar

1½ TB. arrowroot

¾ tsp. aluminum-free baking powder

¾ tsp. baking soda

¾ tsp. gluten-free xanthan gum

¼ tsp. sea salt

3 TB. cold water

1½ TB. Ener-G Egg Replacer

5 TB. vanilla soy milk or other nondairy milk

¼ cup sunflower or other oil

1½ TB. plus 1 tsp. alcohol-free vanilla extract

2¼ tsp. apple cider vinegar

¾ cup seltzer water

⅓ cup nonhydrogenated margarine

3 cups vegan confectioners' sugar

1. Preheat the oven to 350°F. Lightly oil 12 muffin cups (or use paper liners), or use silicone muffin cups.

2. In a large bowl, combine Beverly's Baking Blend, unbleached cane sugar, arrowroot, baking powder, baking soda, xanthan gum, and sea salt.

3. In a small bowl, combine cold water and Ener-G Egg Replacer, and whisk vigorously for 1 minute or until very frothy (like beaten egg whites).

4. Add 3 tablespoons soy milk, sunflower oil, 1½ tablespoons vanilla extract, and apple cider vinegar, and whisk well to combine.

5. Add egg replacer mixture and seltzer water to dry ingredients, and whisk well to combine.

6. Fill prepared muffin cups using a ¼ cup scoop or measuring cup. Bake for 20 to 22 minutes or until a toothpick inserted in the center comes out clean. Remove from the oven. Allow cupcakes to cool slightly in the pan, and transfer to a rack to cool completely before frosting.

7. While cupcakes are cooling, prepare frosting. In a medium bowl, beat margarine with an electric mixer on medium speed or whisk for 30 seconds. Add confectioners' sugar, remaining 2 tablespoons soy milk, and remaining 1 teaspoon vanilla extract, and beat or whisk well for 2 or 3 minutes or until light and fluffy.

8. Using a small spatula, knife, or pastry bag, spread or decoratively pipe frosting on top of each cooled cupcake. Frosted cupcakes are perishable, so we recommend only frosting cupcakes as needed. Store the extra buttercream frosting in an airtight container in the refrigerator and extra unfrosted cupcakes in an airtight plastic container or zipper-lock bag at room temperature.

Variation: If you want to make a colored buttercream frosting, check out the natural tinting suggestions that accompany the Cut-Out Cookies (recipe in Chapter 19). For another nice decorative touch, dip your frosted cupcake into a bowl of vegan multicolored sprinkles or unsweetened shredded coconut. To make a **Frosted Vanilla Cake,** pour the cupcake batter into a lightly oiled 8×10-inch baking pan, or use a silicone baking pan, and bake for 30 to 35 minutes or until a toothpick inserted in the center comes out clean. Allow the cake to cool completely, and frost with the buttercream frosting.

CORNUCOPIA

Many of our baked goods call for seltzer water, which is basically carbonated water, or water into which carbon dioxide gas under pressure has been dissolved. This process causes the water to become effervescent, and the resulting fizzy bubbles act as an additional leavening agent, enabling the other chemical leaveners used in the recipes (such as baking powder or soda) to do their job even better. This helps you get higher and lighter-tasting baked goods.

Pecan Carrot Cake

To make our oil-free carrot cake moist and sweet, we've sweetened it with orange juice and zest, and packed it with shredded carrots, chopped dates, and plump raisins.

Yield:	Prep time:	Cook time:	Serving size:
1 (9-inch) cake or 8 or 9 pieces	15 minutes	40 to 45 minutes	1 piece

¾ cup dried dates, pitted

¾ cup raisins

¾ cup unsweetened coconut water or water

2 cups Bob's Red Mill Gluten-Free All-Purpose Baking Flour

1 tsp. ground cinnamon

1 tsp. ground ginger

¾ tsp. ground cloves or allspice

¾ tsp. freshly grated nutmeg

¾ tsp. aluminum-free baking powder

¾ tsp. baking soda

¾ tsp. gluten-free xanthan gum

¼ tsp. sea salt

1 cup orange juice

2 TB. orange zest

1 TB. apple cider vinegar

2 tsp. alcohol-free vanilla extract

1 cup shredded carrots, slightly packed

⅔ cup raw pecan pieces or roughly chopped pecans

1. Preheat the oven to 375°F. Lightly oil a 9-inch-round (or square) baking pan, or use a silicone baking pan.

2. Cut each date in half lengthwise, and thinly slice crosswise. In a small saucepan, combine cut dates, raisins, and coconut water, and cook over medium heat for 3 minutes. Remove from heat, and set aside to cool slightly.

3. In a medium bowl, combine Bob's Red Mill Gluten-Free All-Purpose Baking Flour, cinnamon, ginger, cloves, nutmeg, baking powder, baking soda, xanthan gum, and sea salt, and whisk well.

4. To date-raisin mixture, stir in orange juice, orange zest, apple cider vinegar, and vanilla extract. Add wet ingredients to dry ingredients, and stir well to combine. Stir in shredded carrots.

5. Transfer batter to the prepared pan. Sprinkle pecans over top, and using your hands, gently press them into cake batter. Bake for 40 to 45 minutes or until a toothpick inserted in the center comes out clean. Remove from the oven, and allow to cool slightly before cutting cake into 8 (for a round cake) or 9 (for a square cake) pieces.

6. Serve warm or at room temperature as desired. Store carrot cake in an airtight container (or cover with plastic wrap) at room temperature.

Variation: You can replace the pecans with an equal amount of roughly chopped walnuts. If you like coconut, add 3 tablespoons unsweetened shredded coconut to the batter when stirring in the shredded carrots. For **Carrot Cupcakes,** portion ¼ cup scoops of batter into lightly oiled muffin cups (or use paper liners) or silicone muffin cups. Evenly sprinkle pecans over individual cupcakes, and bake for 25 to 30 minutes or until a toothpick inserted in the center comes out clean.

MEATLESS AND WHEATLESS

Pecans are one of the most expensive nuts, but most stores tend to put them on sale during the fall and winter seasons. So when you find a good deal, stock up, and freeze them in airtight containers or zipper-lock bags for up to 2 years.

Mini Chocolate Bundt Cakes

Beverly is a self-proclaimed vegan chocoholic, and she was compelled to create these single-serving, rich and chocolaty mini Bundt cakes, covered in After Dark Glaze. Why individual cakes? Because when it comes to chocolate, she doesn't like to share.

Yield:	Prep time:	Cook time:	Serving size:
6 mini Bundt cakes	10 minutes	25 to 30 minutes	1 mini Bundt cake

1 cup Beverly's Baking Blend (recipe in Chapter 3)

¾ cup cocoa powder

¼ cup arrowroot

¾ tsp. gluten-free xanthan gum

¾ tsp. aluminum-free baking powder

½ tsp. ground cinnamon

¼ tsp. plus ⅛ tsp. baking soda

¼ tsp. sea salt

9 TB. maple syrup

9 TB. soy milk or other nondairy milk

½ cup firm or extra-firm silken tofu

6 TB. Prune Paste (variation in Chapter 8)

1½ TB. sunflower oil or other oil

1½ tsp. alcohol-free vanilla extract

¼ tsp. plus ⅛ tsp. apple cider vinegar

1 cup plus 2 TB. After Dark Glaze (recipe earlier in this chapter)

1. Preheat the oven to 350°F. Lightly oil a 6-cavity–mini Bundt cake pan, or use a silicone 6–mini Bundt cake pan.

2. In a large bowl, whisk together Beverly's Baking Blend, cocoa powder, arrowroot, xanthan gum, baking powder, cinnamon, baking soda, and sea salt.

3. In a food processor fitted with an S blade, combine maple syrup, soy milk, silken tofu, Prune Paste, sunflower oil, vanilla extract, and apple cider vinegar, and process for 1 minute or until smooth. Scrape down the sides of the container with a spatula, and process for 30 more seconds.

4. Pour wet ingredients into dry ingredients, and whisk well to combine. Evenly divide batter among the individual Bundt sections of the prepared cake pan.

5. Bake for 25 to 30 minutes or until a toothpick inserted in the center of each Bundt cake comes out clean. Remove from the oven. Let cool in pan for 10 minutes, loosen sides of each Bundt cake with a spatula or knife, and invert onto a rack to cool completely.

6. When Bundt cakes are cool, drizzle 3 tablespoons After Dark Glaze over top of each Bundt cake, and allow it to run down the sides. Glazed Bundt cakes are a bit sticky, so we recommend only glazing these Bundt cakes as needed. Store extra After Dark Glaze in an airtight container in the refrigerator and extra unglazed Bundt cakes in an airtight plastic container or zipper-lock bag at room temperature.

Variation: For a single large **Chocolate Cake,** pour the batter into a lightly oiled 9-inch-round (or square) baking pan, or use a silicone baking pan, and bake for 35 to 40 minutes instead. When the cake has cooled, drizzle the After Dark Glaze over individual servings.

CORNUCOPIA

Bundt cake pans are round with decorated and fluted sides and a tube cut out in the middle to yield a ring-shape cake. Bundt pans are available both in the standard large size and mini. The mini pan contains 6 mini Bundt cake cavities all in one pan, similar to a muffin tin. Silicone Bundt cake pans are widely available as well.

Chocolate Mousse Cake
with Quinoa Crust

If you're still intimidated by gluten-free vegan baking, this decadent, no-bake chocolate mousse cake, which features a surprising cocoa-flavored quinoa base, is for you. The ultracreamy texture resembles a chocolate cheesecake.

Yield:	Prep time:	Cook time:	Serving size:
1 (8-inch) cake or 8 pieces	25 minutes, plus 2 hours or more chill time	25 to 30 minutes	1 piece

½ cup raw pecan pieces or roughly chopped pecans

¾ cup quinoa

2½ cups water

⅓ cup cocoa powder

⅓ cup plus 3 TB. maple syrup

3 tsp. alcohol-free vanilla extract

1 (12-oz.) pkg. vegan gluten-free chocolate chips (about 2 cups)

2 (12-oz.) pkg. extra-firm silken tofu

1. In a medium saucepan, place pecans, and cook over medium heat, shaking saucepan often, for 3 to 5 minutes or until lightly toasted and fragrant. Transfer pecans to a small bowl, and set aside.

2. Place quinoa in a fine mesh sieve, and rinse well under running water for 1 minute. Add water, quinoa, cocoa powder, and ⅓ cup maple syrup to the saucepan, and bring to a boil over high heat. Cover, reduce heat to low, and simmer for 20 to 25 minutes or until quinoa is tender and all liquid is absorbed. Remove from heat.

3. Add 2 teaspoons vanilla extract to quinoa mixture, and stir well. Transfer mixture to a lightly oiled 8-inch springform pan, and spread evenly to cover the bottom of the pan. Every 2 minutes, press down on quinoa mixture with the back of a spoon to compact it into a crust; do this for a total of 10 minutes.

4. Evenly sprinkle half of toasted pecans over quinoa mixture, and set aside.

5. Meanwhile, in the top of a double boiler, place chocolate chips, and heat until thoroughly melted. Remove from heat, and set aside. (Alternatively, place chocolate chips in a microwave-safe bowl and melt in the microwave, heating for 30-second increments until chocolate chips just begin to melt, and stirring until smooth.)

6. In a food processor fitted with an S blade, place silken tofu, melted chocolate chips, remaining 3 tablespoons maple syrup, and remaining 1 teaspoon vanilla extract, and process for 2 minutes. Scrape down the sides of the container with a spatula, and process for 1 more minute or until smooth and creamy.

7. Spread tofu mixture over quinoa crust, and smooth top with a spatula. Evenly sprinkle remaining half of toasted pecans over top. Chill chocolate mousse cake for 2 hours or more or until firm.

8. Loosen sides of cake with a spatula or knife, and remove ring from the springform pan. Cut into 8 pieces, and serve. Cover extra cake with plastic wrap, and store in the refrigerator.

Variation: Feel free to replace the pecans with an equal amount of chopped hazelnuts or almonds, and to further bring out the flavor of the nuts, add $\frac{1}{2}$ teaspoon alcohol-free almond extract to both the quinoa crust and the chocolate mousse filling mixtures. To make a **Mocha Mousse Cake with Quinoa Crust,** prepare the quinoa crust mixture using $1\frac{1}{2}$ cups water and 1 cup regular or decaf coffee, and in the chocolate mousse filling, use only 2 tablespoons maple syrup and $\frac{1}{2}$ teaspoon vanilla extract, and add $1\frac{1}{2}$ tablespoons regular or decaf coffee and $\frac{3}{4}$ teaspoon ground cinnamon.

MEATLESS AND WHEATLESS

It's a myth that you must forsake chocolate as a vegan, although naturally you should avoid milk and most white chocolate selections. Check your local grocery and natural foods store shelves, and you'll likely find many varieties of bittersweet, semi-sweet, white, and dark chocolate bars, chips, and other such products suitable for gluten-free vegans. Don't forget you can also use cocoa powder in your baking, confections, and chocolaty concoctions.

Vegan Cheesecake

We've given commonly used graham crackers the old heave-ho in this cheesecake's crust because most aren't gluten free or vegan. Instead, almond meal is the perfect swap. Our creamy filling is made with silken tofu, vegan cream cheese, a generous amount of vanilla extract, and tart lemon juice and *zest*.

Yield:	Prep time:	Cook time:	Serving size:
1 (8-inch) cake or 8 pieces	25 minutes, plus several hours or more chill time	25 to 30 minutes	1 piece

2 cups almond meal (or an equal amount of finely ground raw almonds)

2 TB. maple syrup

2 TB. sunflower or other oil

1½ tsp. plus 2 TB. alcohol-free vanilla extract

½ tsp. ground cinnamon

¼ tsp. baking soda

2 (8-oz.) pkg. vegan cream cheese

1 (12-oz.) pkg. extra-firm silken tofu

¾ cup unbleached cane sugar

⅓ cup cornstarch

Zest of 2 large lemons

Juice of 2 large lemons

1. Preheat the oven to 350°F. Lightly oil a 8-inch springform pan.

2. In a medium bowl, combine almond meal, maple syrup, sunflower oil, 1½ teaspoons vanilla extract, cinnamon, and baking soda.

3. Transfer crust mixture to the prepared springform pan. Using your hands, firmly press mixture into the bottom of the pan. Bake for 10 minutes or until set. Remove from the oven.

4. Meanwhile, in a food processor fitted with an S blade, place vegan cream cheese, silken tofu, unbleached cane sugar, cornstarch, lemon zest, lemon juice, and remaining 2 tablespoons vanilla extract, and process for 2 minutes. Scrape down the sides of the container with a spatula, and process for 1 or 2 more minutes or until smooth and creamy.

5. Spread tofu mixture over prebaked crust, and smooth top with a spatula. Bake for 45 to 50 more minutes or until set. Remove from the oven.

6. Let cheesecake cool for 15 minutes, and use a spatula or knife to loosen cheese-cake from the sides of the springform pan. Place cheesecake on a rack to cool to room temperature. Chill cheesecake for several hours or overnight, or until firm.

7. Again, loosen sides of cheesecake with a spatula or knife, and remove ring from the springform pan. Cut cheesecake into 8 pieces, and serve. Cover extra cheesecake with plastic wrap, and store in the refrigerator.

Variation: This recipe makes a plain, lemon-vanilla cheesecake, but if you're so inclined, you can dress up your finished cheesecake in several ways, such as topping it with whole or sliced fresh fruit or berries or drizzling a little melted chocolate over the top.

DEFINITION

Zest is the colorful outer peel of lemons, limes, oranges, and other citrus fruits. It contains the aromatic essential oils of the fruit, so it beneficially adds a concentrated citrus flavor without adding a lot of excess moisture to foods. You can easily remove the zest from a citrus fruit using a zester or fine or Microplane grater.

Glossary

agar powder (or **agar-agar flakes**)   An odorless, tasteless powder derived from a variety of seaweed that can be used as a vegan replacement for gelatin (which is an animal-based by-product).

al dente   Italian for "against the teeth." Refers to pasta or rice that's neither soft nor hard, but just slightly firm against the teeth.

allspice   Named for its flavor echoes of several spices (cinnamon, cloves, nutmeg), allspice is used in many desserts and in rich marinades and stews.

almonds   Mild, sweet, and crunchy nuts that combine nicely with creamy and sweet food items.

alpha-linolenic acid   An omega-3 fatty acid found in plants (chiefly in seed oils) that ultimately can be converted into EPA and then DHA.

amandine   A French culinary term that indicates that the final dish has a garnish of whole, sliced, or toasted almonds. It's often erroneously spelled as *almondine*.

antioxidants   Vitamins, minerals, and phytonutrients that slow or stop the process of oxidation, which is what leads to aging and chronic disease development.

arborio rice   A plump Italian rice used, among other purposes, for risotto.

arrowroot   A gluten-free thickener, more stable than flour to temperature and acidity, that maintains a neutral taste and clear color and provides a transparent sheen.

artichoke hearts   The center part of the artichoke flower, often found canned in grocery stores.

arugula   A spicy-peppery garden plant with leaves that resemble a dandelion and have a distinctive—and very sharp—flavor.

autoimmune disease   Any condition (including type 1 diabetes, lupus, and multiple sclerosis) that results in the body's immune system mistakenly attacking itself, leading to self-perpetuating symptom progression.

bake   To cook in a dry oven. Dry-heat cooking often results in a crisping of the exterior of the food being cooked. Moist-heat cooking, through methods such as steaming, poaching, etc., brings a much different, moist quality to the food.

baking powder   A dry ingredient used to increase volume and lighten or leaven baked goods. It's made of the alkaline substance baking soda (sodium bicarbonate), an acid (like cream of tartar), and an inert starch to absorb the moisture.

barbecue   To quick-cook over high heat, or to cook something long and slow in a rich liquid (barbecue sauce).

basil   A flavorful, almost sweet, resinous herb delicious with tomatoes and used in all kinds of Italian- or Mediterranean-style dishes.

baste   To keep foods moist during cooking by spooning, brushing, or drizzling with a liquid.

beat   To quickly mix substances.

black forbidden rice   A short-grain heirloom rice variety that has a deep, purplish-black color and a slightly nutty flavor. It was originally cultivated exclusively for the emperors of China.

blanch   To place a food in boiling water for about 1 minute (or less) to partially cook the exterior and then submerge in or rinse with cool water to halt the cooking.

blend   To completely mix something, usually with a blender or food processor, more slowly than beating.

boil   To heat a liquid to a point where water is forced to turn into steam, causing the liquid to bubble. To boil something is to insert it into boiling water. A rapid boil is when a lot of bubbles form on the surface of the liquid.

Bragg Liquid Aminos   Made from soybeans and water, with a salty, rich flavor similar to tamari or other soy sauce. It is commonly used as a condiment and flavor enhancer and contains large amounts of dietary essential and nonessential amino acids.

broil   To cook in a dry oven under the overhead high-heat element.

brown rice   Whole-grain rice including the germ with a characteristic pale brown or tan color; more nutritious and flavorful than white rice.

buckwheat flour   Made by finely grinding buckwheat groats, it is neither a grain nor a grass, but rather a fruit seed, and a member of the rhubarb family of plants. Although it might sound like a type of wheat, buckwheat is not related to wheat at all.

caraway   A distinctive spicy seed used for bread and cabbage dishes. It's known to reduce stomach upset, which is why it's often paired with, for example, sauerkraut.

cardamom   An intense, sweet-smelling spice, common to Indian cooking, used in baking and coffee.

carnival squash   Small, pumpkin-shape squashes that come in several shades, such as pale yellow to cream color with orange, pale green, or dark green spots or vertical stripes. Their flavor is often compared to a sweet potato or butternut squash.

carob   A tropical tree that produces long pods. The dried, baked, and powdered flesh (carob powder) is used in baking, and the fresh and dried pods are used for a variety of recipes. The flavor is sweet and reminiscent of chocolate.

carotenoids   A category of up to hundreds of naturally occurring organic pigments in plants with red, orange, and yellow hues. Several have potent antioxidant properties.

cayenne   A fiery spice made from (hot) chile peppers, especially the cayenne chile, a slender, red, and very hot pepper.

celiac disease   Another term for celiac sprue, an autoimmune condition that damages the lining of the small intestines and leads to nutritional deficiencies and other chronic illnesses when gluten is consumed.

chickpea (or **garbanzo bean**)   Yellow-gold, roundish beans used as the base ingredient in hummus. Chickpeas are high in fiber and low in fat.

chickpea flour   Flour made from dried chickpeas that have been finely ground to a flourlike consistency. Chickpea flour is used to replace wheat in gluten-free cooking and baking due to its high protein content. It is also referred to as garbanzo bean, besan, or gram flour, and is often used in Middle Eastern, Indian, and African cuisines.

chiffonade   French for "made from rags," a technique for slicing herbs and vegetables into long, thin, ribbonlike strips. This reference is usually applied to leaves of basil, mint, or leafy green vegetables. To chiffonade something, stack and roll a small pile of leaves; slice the roll crosswise into fine, thin strips; and gently toss the strips with your fingers to separate them.

chile (or **chili**)   Any one of many different "hot" peppers, ranging in intensity from the relatively mild ancho pepper to the blisteringly hot habañero.

chili powder   A seasoning blend that includes chile pepper, cumin, garlic, and oregano. Proportions vary among different versions, but they all offer a warm, rich flavor.

Chinese five-spice powder   A seasoning blend of cinnamon, anise, ginger, fennel, and pepper.

chop   To cut into pieces, usually qualified by an adverb such as "*coarsely* chopped," or by a size measurement such as "chopped into $\frac{1}{2}$-inch pieces." "Finely chopped" is much closer to mince.

cilantro   A member of the parsley family used in Mexican cooking (especially salsa) and some Asian dishes. Use in moderation, as the flavor can overwhelm. The seed of the cilantro plant is the spice coriander.

cinnamon   A rich, aromatic spice commonly used in baking or desserts. Cinnamon can also be used for delicious and interesting entrées.

clabbering   A process done by combining soy milk (or other nondairy) with a little lemon juice or vinegar, which when left to sit for a few minutes, will cause the soy milk to sour and thicken slightly. Sometimes this mixture is referred to as soy buttermilk because it can be used as a measure-for-measure replacement for buttermilk in recipes.

clove   A sweet, strong, almost wintergreen-flavor spice used in baking.

coconut water   The clear to translucent liquid found inside a young green coconut. It's mild and sweet in flavor and rich in electrolytes, making it the perfect natural sports drink.

coriander   A rich, warm, spicy seed used in all types of cuisines, from African to South American, and dishes from entrées to desserts.

cornstarch   One of the most commonly used starches in baking and food processing. Essentially, it's the refined starch of the endosperm of the corn kernel. Cornstarch functions as a vegan, gluten-free thickener and is also often mixed with cold liquid to make into a paste before adding to a recipe to avoid clumps.

crimini mushrooms   A relative of the white button mushroom but brown in color and with a richer flavor. The larger, fully grown version is the portobello. *See also* portobello mushrooms.

cross-reactivity   A condition where your body's immune system mistakes other food proteins for ones you can't tolerate and creates an autoimmune reaction to them, making you react to these other foods in the same way as you would gluten.

crudités   Fresh vegetables served as an appetizer, often all together on one tray.

cumin   A fiery, smoky-tasting spice popular in Middle Eastern and Indian dishes. Cumin is a seed; ground cumin seed is the most common form used in cooking.

curry   Rich, spicy, Indian-style sauces and the dishes prepared with them. A curry uses curry powder as its base seasoning.

curry powder   A ground blend of rich and flavorful spices used as a basis for curry and many other Indian-influenced dishes. Common ingredients include hot pepper, nutmeg, cumin, cinnamon, pepper, and turmeric. Some curry can also be found in paste form.

dash   A few drops, usually of a liquid, released by a quick shake of, for example, a bottle of hot sauce.

demerara sugar   A large, coarsely granulated variety of cane sugar that hails from the Demerara region of Guyana. It has a golden amber color and slight molasses flavor and can be used as a replacement for light or dark brown sugar in recipes.

DHA   Docosahexaenoic acid, an omega-3 fatty acid thought to be important for infant brain, eye, and nerve cell development.

dice   To cut into small cubes about $\frac{1}{4}$-inch square.

Dietary Reference Intakes (DRI)   Nutritional guidelines for optimal levels of carbohydrates, protein, fat, vitamins, and minerals set by the Institute of Medicine's Food and Nutrition Board.

dill   A herb perfect for vegetables (pickles!).

dollop   A spoonful of something creamy and thick.

double boiler   A set of two pots designed to nest together, one inside the other, and provide consistent, moist heat for foods that need delicate treatment. The bottom pot holds water (not quite touching the bottom of the top pot); the top pot holds the ingredient you want to heat.

dredge   To cover a piece of food with a dry substance such as flour or cornmeal.

drizzle   To lightly sprinkle drops of a liquid over food, often as the finishing touch to a dish.

edamame   Pale green, plump, fresh soybeans, similar in appearance to lima beans. You can typically find them prepackaged, both shelled or still in their protective pods, in the freezer section.

EPA   Eicosapentaenoic acid, an omega-3 fatty acid.

escarole   A variety of endive that has very broad, bitter-tasting leaves. A medium head of escarole usually yields about 7 cups torn leaves. It can be eaten raw in salads, blanched or boiled in water, or sautéed.

extra-virgin olive oil   *See* olive oil.

fennel   In seed form, a fragrant, licorice-tasting herb. The bulbs have a much milder flavor and a celerylike crunch and are used as a vegetable in salads or cooked recipes.

flax eggs   A phenomenal answer to baking and cooking egg free. They look, taste, act, and feel like egg whites, yet they're healthy (omega-3 fatty acids), much less expensive, and work just as well. For an equivalent of 1 egg, combine 1 tablespoon ground flaxseeds or flaxseed meal to 3 tablespoons water, blend or whisk, and allow to sit for 5 minutes.

floret   The flower or bud end of broccoli or cauliflower.

flour   Grains ground into a meal. Wheat is perhaps the most common flour. Flour is also made from gluten-free grains, nuts, and legumes such as brown rice, buck-wheat, amaranth, quinoa, fava beans, chickpeas, soybeans, etc.

flute   To give a decorative edge to a piecrust by pressing or pinching the pastry with your fingers or the tines of a fork.

fold   To combine a dense and light mixture with a circular action from the middle of the bowl.

fry   *See* sauté.

garam masala   Literally "hot spice" in Hindi. Garam masala is made with a blend of pungent and warming spices and doesn't necessarily have a hot flavor like cayenne or chile powder. The flavorful blend is commonly used in Indian and Southern Asian cuisines as an alternative to curry powder, and although blends vary by brand, most contain cardamom, cinnamon, coriander, cumin, cloves, and black pepper.

garlic   A member of the onion family, a pungent and flavorful element in many savory dishes. A garlic bulb contains multiple cloves. Each clove, when chopped, provides about 1 teaspoon garlic. Most recipes call for cloves or chopped garlic by the teaspoon.

ginger   Available in fresh root or dried, ground form, ginger adds a pungent, sweet, and spicy quality to a dish.

golden flaxseeds   The pale yellow sister of the more commonly used nutty brown flaxseeds. Both forms of flaxseeds can be used interchangeably on foods and in baked goods, but because they're lighter in color, the golden flaxseeds are less visible in baked goods, which can be advantageous in light-colored cookie and cake batters.

gomasio   A condiment made from dry roasted sesame seeds that have been ground together with a little sea salt. It can be used as a condiment on noodles, rice, and other cooked grains; miso soup; stir-fries; and other Asian dishes in place of sesame seeds. It can also be used as a tasty seasoning and a replacement for table salt.

grate   To shave into tiny pieces using a sharp rasp or grater.

grind   To reduce a large, hard substance, often a seasoning such as peppercorns, to the consistency of sand.

guar gum   A soluble fiber that thickens tremendously when mixed with water and contributes to viscosity, helps maintain stability, and acts as an emulsifier.

handful   An unscientific measurement; the amount of an ingredient you can hold in your hand.

hazelnuts (also **filberts**)   A sweet nut popular in desserts and, to a lesser degree, savory dishes.

heirloom tomatoes   Tomatoes cultivated using seeds that have been passed down from generation to generation and are prized by growers and consumers for their exceptional flavor. They can be found in a wide variety of green, yellow, orange, pink, red, red-brown, purple-black, and even striped colors; in round, elongated, and bulging shapes of various sizes; and with flavors that range from sweet or savory to slightly bitter.

herbes de Provence   A seasoning mix including basil, fennel, marjoram, rosemary, sage, and thyme, common in the south of France.

Himalayan pink salt   A hand-mined salt derived from ancient sea salt deposits found in the Himalayan Mountains and considered by some to be the purest variety of salt available. The salt crystals range in color from sheer white, to varying shades of pink, to deep reds due to its high mineral and iron content.

hors d'oeuvre   French for "outside of work" (the "work" being the main meal), an hors d'oeuvre can be any dish served as a starter before the meal.

horseradish A sharp, spicy root that forms the flavor base in many condiments from cocktail sauce to sharp mustards. Prepared horseradish contains vinegar and oil, among other ingredients. Use pure horseradish much more sparingly than the prepared version, or try cutting it with vegan sour cream.

hummus A thick, Middle Eastern spread made of puréed garbanzo beans, lemon juice, olive oil, garlic, and often tahini (sesame seed paste).

Italian seasoning A blend of dried herbs, including basil, oregano, rosemary, and thyme.

jicama A juicy, crunchy, sweet, large, round Central American vegetable. If you can't find jicama, try substituting sliced water chestnuts.

julienne A French word meaning "to slice into very thin pieces." Here's how: after washing and peeling your vegetable, cut a flat surface on each of the vegetable's four sides, making a rectangle shape. Next, cut $\frac{1}{8}$-inch slices through the vegetable. Finally, stack the rectangles flat on top of one another and repeat the $\frac{1}{8}$-inch slices again, until you have thin matchsticklike strips.

kalamata olives Traditionally from Greece, these medium-small long black olives have a smoky rich flavor.

Key limes Very small limes grown primarily in Florida known for their tart taste.

knead To work dough to make it pliable so it holds gas bubbles as it bakes. Kneading is fundamental in the process of making yeast breads.

kosher salt A coarse-grained salt made without any additives or iodine.

lacinato kale An heirloom variety of kale that has tender, dark blue-green leaves, that have a slightly sweeter and more delicate taste than curly green kale. It's also referred to as Tuscan, Italian, or comically as dinosaur kale because the extremely wrinkled leaves have a somewhat prehistoric look.

lemongrass A thick, lemon-scented grass commonly used in Thai dishes. When buying fresh lemongrass, look for stalks that are fragrant, tightly formed, and lemony-green colored, or for an easier preparation, purchase lemongrass that comes in a jar with water.

lentils Tiny lens-shape pulses used in European, Middle Eastern, and Indian cuisines.

maitake mushrooms Wild mushrooms that have a rich woodsy flavor and have small, overlapping, fan-shape caps. The name literally translates from Japanese as "dancing mushroom." They're also known as "hen of the woods."

marjoram   A sweet herb, a cousin of and similar to oregano, popular in Greek, Spanish, and Italian dishes.

Microplane   A handheld grater that can be used to finely grate cheeses, chocolate, and vegetables, and also to remove the zest from citrus fruits.

millet   A tiny, round, yellow-colored grain native to Africa. It has a nutty flavor and is often used as a replacement for couscous because it has a similar appearance and texture. It can be enjoyed as a grain side dish or added whole or ground into flour for use in making breads and baked goods.

mince   To cut into very small pieces smaller than diced pieces, about $\frac{1}{8}$ inch or smaller.

miso   A fermented, flavorful soybean paste, key in many Japanese dishes.

mochi (pronounced *mo-chee*)   A Japanese rice snack made from sweet short-grain brown rice that's been steamed and pounded, mashed, or finely ground and then allowed to cool before being shaped into blocks. Mochi has a slightly chewy texture when baked and can be enjoyed as a snack, or used for preparing sweet or savory recipes.

mousse   A light and creamy puddinglike dessert. In classic French cooking, a mousse is often prepared with a mixture of heavy cream, beaten eggs (or just egg whites), dissolved gelatin, sugar, and/or melted chocolate, fruit purées, or other flavoring ingredients. In contrast, the base of a vegan mousse is typically prepared using blended tofu, soy creamer, or nondairy milks, which are then combined with a thickening agent, sweetener, and other ingredients. *Mousse* in French means "lather" or "foam."

nutmeg   A sweet, fragrant, musky spice used primarily in baking.

nutritional yeast flakes   An inactive yeast that has a nutty, almost cheeselike flavor, which is why it's commonly used as an imitation cheese flavoring for foods and in the production of nondairy cheese products. It's an excellent product for vegans to use to attain their recommended daily dose of vitamin B_{12}. Do not confuse with active yeast, the type used for making breads and baked goods.

olive oil   A fragrant liquid produced by crushing or pressing olives. Extra-virgin olive oil—the most flavorful and highest quality—is produced from the first pressing of a batch of olives; oil is also produced from later pressings.

olives   The fruit of the olive tree commonly grown on all sides of the Mediterranean. Black olives are also called ripe olives. Green olives are immature, although they're also widely eaten. *See also* kalamata olives.

omega-3 fatty acids   A family of essential polyunsaturated fat found in flax, hemp, chia, soybeans, tofu, leafy green vegetables, and walnuts. They provide health benefits, including anti-inflammatory, immune-enhancing, and cardio-protective effects.

omega-6 fatty acids   A group of essential polyunsaturated fats widely available in many dietary sources, especially vegetable oils. Although these are essential, in high doses (common in Western societies), they promote inflammation and disease. A lower ratio of omega-6:omega-3 fatty acids is optimal.

oregano   A fragrant, slightly astringent herb used in Greek, Spanish, and Italian dishes.

oxidation   The browning of fruit flesh that happens over time and with exposure to air. Minimize oxidation by rubbing the cut surfaces with lemon juice.

paprika   A rich, red, warm, earthy spice that lends a rich red color to many dishes.

parboil   To partially cook in boiling water or broth, similar to blanching (although blanched foods are quickly cooled with cold water).

parsley   A fresh-tasting green leafy herb, often used as a garnish.

pâté   A savory loaf or spread served cold on crusty bread or crackers.

pecans   Rich, buttery nuts, native to North America, that have a high unsaturated fat content.

peppercorns   Large, round, dried berries ground to produce pepper.

phytonutrients   Naturally occurring plant compounds that confer health benefits, including performing antioxidant, anti-inflammatory, antiseptic, and/or a host of other activities.

pickle   A food, usually a vegetable such as a cucumber, that's been pickled in brine.

pilaf   A rice dish in which the rice is browned in butter or oil and then cooked in a flavorful liquid such as a broth, often with the addition of vegetables. The rice absorbs the broth, resulting in a savory dish.

pinch   An unscientific measurement term, the amount of an ingredient—typically a dry, granular substance such as an herb or seasoning—you can hold between your finger and thumb.

pine nuts (also **pignoli** or **piñon**)   Nuts grown on pine trees that are rich (read: high fat), flavorful, and a bit piney. Pine nuts are a traditional component of pesto and add a wonderful hearty crunch to many other recipes.

poach   To cook a food in simmering liquid, such as water, wine, or broth.

portobello mushrooms   A mature and larger form of the smaller crimini mushroom, portobellos are brownish, chewy, and flavorful. Often served as whole caps, grilled, and as thin sautéed slices. *See also* crimini mushrooms.

pot liquor (pot likker)   The nutritious and flavorful liquid that accumulates from cooking vegetables, most notably green leafy vegetables. It's customary to sop up your pot liquor with pieces of bread, cornbread, or biscuits.

potato starch   A starch used as a thickener, especially in soups, gravies, stews, and sauces. It's also a gluten-free vegan way to add moistness in baking.

poultry seasoning blend   A blend of dried herbs and spices, which often includes sage, thyme, rosemary, marjoram, black pepper, and celery seed. It's so named because many of these seasonings are used to flavor poultry, but it can also be used as a seasoning for stuffing, rice, and grains, as well as vegetable-based dishes.

powdered kelp   Made from cleaned and sun-dried kelp, a type of seaweed (or sea vegetable). Adding a little powdered kelp or other sea vegetables to your dishes imparts a slightly fishy flavor, which is why they're commonly added to mock fish dishes, like vegan pâté or tuna salad.

preheat   To turn on an oven, broiler, or other cooking appliance in advance of cooking so the temperature will be at the desired level when the assembled dish is ready for cooking.

prepared horseradish   Grated horseradish root that's been preserved in vinegar, or bottled with beet juice as in the case of red horseradish, and is sold in small glass jars or bottles in the refrigerated section of most stores. Check the ingredient label carefully to be sure it isn't actually horseradish sauce because that condiment often contains eggs or dairy-based products.

probiotics   Live microorganisms that, when consumed in adequate quantities, confer health benefits on the host, including improved immunity and digestion.

pseudocereal   Broadleaf plants (nongrasses) used in similar ways as cereals (usually grasses), such as amaranth, quinoa, and buckwheat.

purée   To reduce a food to a thick, creamy texture, usually using a blender or food processor.

quinoa flakes   Quinoa that's been prewashed (to remove the bitter and protective saponin coating) and then steamrolled into a quick-cooking flake. You can enjoy quinoa flakes cooked in liquid for a hot cereal, or use them as a replacement for rolled oats in baked goods.

rapid-rise active yeast   A variety of baker's yeast that's essentially an instant version of active dry yeast. It must be hydrated to activate the dough and cause the rise to occur.

raw cacao powder   A powder made from raw cacao beans that have gone through a cold-pressing process to remove the fat (cacao butter) and are then finely ground into a powder, much like cocoa powder (which is made from roasted cacao beans). It has a deep, dark, almost coffeelike flavor and is often used by raw foodists and others as a replacement for cocoa powder in recipes.

raw vanilla bean powder   Made by grinding whole, dried vanilla beans. It has a very intense flavor; $\frac{1}{2}$ teaspoon vanilla bean powder is the equivalent of 1 teaspoon vanilla extract.

reduce   To boil or simmer a broth or sauce to remove some of the water content, resulting in more concentrated flavor and color.

reserve   To hold a specified ingredient for another use later in the recipe.

rice vinegar   Vinegar produced from fermented rice or rice wine, popular in Asian-style dishes. Different from rice wine vinegar.

roast   To cook something uncovered in an oven, usually without additional liquid.

rosemary   A pungent, sweet herb. A little of it goes a long way.

saffron   A spice made from the stamens of crocus flowers, saffron lends a dramatic yellow color and distinctive flavor to a dish. Use only tiny amounts of this expensive herb.

sage   An herb with a musty yet fruity lemon-rind scent and "sunny" flavor.

salsa   A style of mixing fresh vegetables and/or fresh fruit in a coarse chop. Salsa can be spicy or not, fruit-based or not, and served as a starter on its own (with chips, for example) or as a companion to a main course.

salt   A seasoning used in baked goods to enhance flavor, help strengthen the protein in dough, and steady the fermentation rate. Because it provides functional support to baked goods and works as part of the chemical reactions, it's necessary to include it in those recipes.

saturated fat Fat that's solid at room temperature, mostly found in animal products, but also in the plant world from tropical oils like coconut, palm, and palm kernel oil. Saturated fat is completely unnecessary in the diet.

sauté To pan-cook over lower heat than used for frying.

savory A popular herb with a fresh, woody taste.

sear To quickly brown the exterior of a food over high heat to preserve interior moisture.

shallot A member of the onion family that grows in a bulb somewhat like garlic and has a milder onion flavor. When a recipe calls for shallot, use the entire bulb.

shiitake mushrooms Large, dark brown mushrooms with a hearty, meaty flavor. Can be used fresh, dried, or grilled; as a component in other recipes; and as a flavoring source for broth.

short-grain rice A starchy rice popular for Asian-style dishes because it readily clumps—perfect for eating with chopsticks.

shred To cut into many long, thin slices.

silken tofu Made from soybeans and has a velvety-smooth and creamy texture. The process for making silken tofu differs slightly from regular tofu, in that the soy milk curds and excess water are not separated during production. Depending on the silken tofu's final texture, it's labeled soft, firm, or extra-firm. Silken tofu is often blended for making sauces, salad dressings, beverages, desserts, and baked goods.

Silpat liners Reusable, nonstick baking mats made of fiberglass and silicone that are often used to line cookie sheets and baking pans as an alternative to lightly oiling or using parchment paper.

simmer To boil gently so the liquid barely bubbles.

skillet (also **frying pan**) A generally heavy, flat-bottomed metal pan with a handle designed to cook food over heat on a stovetop.

slice To cut into thin pieces.

smoked paprika A variety of Spanish paprika. Smoked paprika is made from mature pimento peppers that are dried; naturally smoked over oak wood fires; and stone-ground to a fine, powdery consistency. It has a deep red color, with a slightly smoky and bittersweet flavor.

smoked sea salt   Sea salt that's been slow-smoked for several hours over various types of wood, such as hickory, mesquite, or alder. It has a full-bodied, very intense, smoky flavor and aroma and is often used as a replacement for liquid smoke flavoring to add a bit of smokiness to barbecue sauces, marinades, dry rubs, and grilled or oven-roasted items.

sorghum (milo)   A cereal grass cultivated to make flour or for use as a feed grain. Nutritionally dense with fiber, iron, phosphorus, potassium, calcium, and protein, sorghum adds volume, texture, crumb, and a slightly nutty flavor to baked goods.

sorghum syrup (sorghum molasses)   Made from the sweet sorghum variety of the cereal grain sorghum. In a process similar to making molasses from sugarcane, the sweet juices that have been extracted from the plants' stalks are boiled down to create mild-flavored, amber-colored syrup.

spiralizer (spiral slicer)   A kitchen gadget that quickly and easily creates spiral strands, curly ribbons, or paper-thin slices of fruits and vegetables.

steam   To suspend a food over boiling water and allow the heat of the steam (water vapor) to cook the food. A quick-cooking method, steaming preserves the flavor and texture of a food.

stew   To slowly cook pieces of food submerged in a liquid. Also, a dish that has been prepared by this method.

stir-fry   To cook small pieces of food in a wok or skillet over high heat, moving and turning the food quickly to cook all sides.

super firm tofu   Tofu that's had most of the water pressed out of it prior to packaging, which gives the block of tofu an extremely dense texture. Super firm tofu can be used in many dishes, especially in recipes that call for marinating, grilling, baking, or frying the tofu.

tahini   A paste made from sesame seeds used to flavor many Middle Eastern recipes.

tapioca pearls   Made from tapioca starch (a.k.a. tapioca flour) that's soaked, cooked, shaped, and dried into assorted sizes of pellets or pearls.

tapioca starch   Originating from the cassava root, a starchy tuber that resembles a potato. In dough, tapioca gelatinizes during baking and adds chewiness to the texture. This also enables the finished product to maintain structure.

tarragon   A sweet, rich-smelling herb perfect with vegetables, especially asparagus.

tart pan   Used for baking both quiches and sweet and savory tarts, which in contrast to slope-sided pie pans, have fluted or straight sides. Many tart pans also feature a removable bottom and outer ring construction, which makes for easier transferring of the finished tart or quiche to a plate or cake stand for serving.

thyme   A minty, zesty herb.

toasted buckwheat groats (kasha)   Buckwheat groats that have been roasted to give them a slightly nutty aroma and flavor. They can be cooked in water or another liquid for eating as a hot cereal or used in making vanishkas, pilafs, knishes, and blintzes.

toasted sesame oil   An oil, made from pressing toasted sesame seeds, that's very aromatic and flavorful, and often used in Asian cuisine.

tofu   A cheeselike substance made from soybeans and soy milk.

tomatillos   Small, round, pale-green fruits of the tomatillo plant that grow enclosed in a protective, paperlike husk. They have a tart flavor and much firmer texture than tomatoes, which they're often confused with.

trans fat   Fat that's possibly worse for your health than saturated fat. It's created in a lab via a process called hydrogenation and used to extend shelf life. It's found primarily in margarine, highly processed, and fried food products.

turbinado sugar   Sugar made from the juice extracted from unrefined raw cane sugar, which is then spun in a centrifuge or turbine (hence its name). It has a very fine texture and a slight molasses flavor. It can also be used to replace light brown sugar. You might be familiar with the most commonly sold brand of turbinado sugar—Sugar in the Raw.

turmeric   A spicy, pungent yellow root used in many dishes, especially Indian cuisine, for color and flavor. Turmeric is the source of the yellow color in many prepared mustards.

vegetable steamer   An insert for a large saucepan, or a special pot with tiny holes in the bottom designed to fit on another pot, to hold food to be steamed above boiling water. *See also* steam.

villi   Tiny, fingerlike projections found along the small intestine that increase the surface area, enabling absorption of nutrients from digested food into the bloodstream.

vinegar   An acidic liquid widely used as dressing and seasoning, often made from fermented grapes, apples, or rice. *See also* rice vinegar; white vinegar.

walnuts   Rich, slightly woody-flavored nuts.

wasabi (or wasabi powder)   Japanese horseradish, a fiery, pungent condiment used with many Japanese-style dishes. It's most often sold as a powder, and you add water to create a paste.

water chestnuts   A tuber, popular in many types of Asian-style cooking. The flesh is white, crunchy, and juicy, and the vegetable holds its texture whether cool or hot.

watermelon daikon radishes   Radishes that are round like a beet and have a similar appearance to their namesake with a light green outer skin and bright pink inside. They're unlike a daikon radish, which looks like a long, overly fat, large white carrot.

whisk   To rapidly mix, introducing air to the mixture.

white mushrooms   Button mushrooms. When fresh, they have an earthy smell and an appealing soft crunch.

wild rice   Actually a grass with a rich, nutty flavor, popular as an unusual and nutritious side dish.

wok   A round-bottomed cooking vessel, originating in China, that's typically used for stir-frying, braising, steaming, stewing, deep frying, and making soup because it evenly distributes heat and enables easy tossing of ingredients.

xanthan gum   Similar to guar gum in its characteristics and uses and made from a microorganism called *Xanthomonas campestris*, it's effective at thickening, stabilizing, and emulsifying dressings and sauces in tiny amounts and providing the gumminess in dough when used in baking.

yeast   Tiny fungi that, when mixed with water, sugar, flour, and heat, release carbon dioxide bubbles, which, in turn, cause the bread to rise.

zest   Small slivers of peel, usually from citrus fruits such as lemon, lime, or orange.

zester   A kitchen tool used to scrape zest off a fruit. A small grater or Microplane also works well.

Resources

As you can see from the books, products, and other information in this appendix, a wide world of resources is available to help support your gluten-free vegan lifestyle. Specialty food items, health experts, and national organizations flood the Internet and you are only a click away from answers to your questions, concerns, and needs. A vastly growing library of literature is also available and will further empower you to make healthy and compassionate choices.

Gluten-Free and Vegan Products

Barry Farm Foods
barryfarm.com
Unsweetened carob chips

Bob's Red Mill
bobsredmill.com
Gluten-free flours, starches, grains, etc.

Cosmo's Vegan Shoppe
cosmosveganshoppe.com

Dragünara
dragunara.com
Spices and sauces

Ener-G Foods
ener-G.com

Enjoy Life Natural Brands
enjoylifefoods.com
Gluten-free, dairy-free, nut-free, and other allergen-free products

Follow Your Heart
followyourheart.com
Vegan cheeses, cream cheese, sour cream, Vegenaise, and salad dressings

Food for Life
foodforlife.com
Tons of good gluten-free breads, English muffins, and other such products

The Gluten-Free Mall
glutenfreemall.com

LocalHarvest
localharvest.org/csa
Locate and join your local CSA

Lundberg Family Farms
lundberg.com

Mountain Rose Herbs
mountainroseherbs.com

Organics Are for Everyone
organicsareforeveryone.com
Date syrup

Quinoa Corporation/Ancient Harvest
quinoa.net
Quinoa, quinoa flakes, and polenta

SunSpire
sunspire.com
Vegan chocolate chips

Turtle Mountain
turtlemountain.com
Lots of yummy vegan nondairy milks, ice cream, yogurt, etc.—even gluten-free cookie dough

VeganEssentials
veganessentials.com

Vitacost.com
vitacost.com

Wildwood
wildwoodfoods.com
Tofu (especially sprouted and super firm), soy-based products, and yogurt

YC Chocolate
ycchocolate.com
Gluten-free, vegan, sugar-free dark chocolate bars

Gluten-Free Information and Support

American Celiac Disease Alliance
americanceliac.org

Celiac Disease Foundation
celiac.org

Celiac Sprue Association
csaceliacs.org

Children's Digestive Health and Nutrition Foundation
cdhnf.org

Gluten Intolerance Group of North America
gluten.net

National Digestive Diseases Information Clearinghouse
digestive.niddk.nih.gov/ddiseases/pubs/celiac

National Foundation for Celiac Awareness
celiaccentral.org

Vegan Information and Support

American Dietetic Association's Vegetarian Group
vegetariannutrition.net

Beverly Lynn Bennett
veganchef.com

Brenda Davis, R.D.
brendadavisrd.com

Dr. Joel Fuhrman
drfuhrman.com

Dr. McDougall's Health and Medical Center
drmcdougall.com

HappyCow
happycow.net
Plant-based dining options

John Robbins
johnrobbins.info

Physicians Committee for Responsible Medicine (PCRM)
pcrm.org

The Plant-Based Dietitian
plantbaseddietitian.com
toyourhealthnutrition.blogspot.com

T. Colin Campbell Foundation
tcolincampbell.org

TrueNorth Health Center
healthpromoting.com

Vegetarian Resource Group
vrg.org

Vegetarians in Paradise
vegparadise.com

VegNews **magazine**
vegnews.com

VegSource
vegsource.com

Books

Anderson, Mike. *The RAVE Diet and Lifestyle, Third Edition.* RaveDiet.com, 2009.

Barnard, Neal D. *21-Day Weight Loss Kickstart: Boost Metabolism, Lower Cholesterol, and Dramatically Improve Your Health.* New York: Grand Central Life and Style, 2011.

————. *Breaking the Food Seduction: The Hidden Reasons Behind Food Cravings—and 7 Steps to End Them Naturally.* New York: St. Martin's Griffin, 2004.

Bennett, Beverly Lynn. *Vegan Bites: Recipes for Singles.* Summertown, PA: Book Publishing Company, 2008.

Bennett, Beverly Lynn, and Ray Sammartano. *The Complete Idiot's Guide to Vegan Cooking.* Indianapolis: Alpha Books, 2008.

————. *The Complete Idiot's Guide to Vegan Living.* Indianapolis: Alpha Books, 2005.

Campbell, T. Colin, and Thomas M. Campbell II. *The China Study: The Most Comprehensive Study of Nutrition Ever Conducted and The Startling Implications for Diet, Weight Loss and Long-Term Health.* Dallas: BenBella Books, 2006.

Chef AJ. *Unprocessed*. Los Angeles: Hail to the Kale Publishing, 2011.

Davis, Brenda, and Vesanto Melina. *Becoming Raw: The Essential Guide to Raw Vegan Diets*. Summertown, TN: Book Publishing Company, 2010.

———. *Becoming Vegan*. Summertown, TN: Book Publishing Company, 2000.

Esselstyn Jr., Caldwell B. *Prevent and Reverse Heart Disease: The Revolutionary, Scientifically Proven, Nutrition-Based Cure*. New York: Penguin Group, 2007.

Esselstyn, Rip. *The Engine 2 Diet: The Texas Firefighter's 28-Day Save-Your-Life Plan That Lowers Cholesterol and Burns Away the Pounds*. New York: Wellness Central, 2009.

Freedman, Rory, and Kim Barnouin. *Skinny Bitch*. Philadelphia: Running Press, 2005.

Fuhrman, Joel. *Eat to Live: The Amazing Nutrient-Rich Program for Fast and Sustained Weight Loss*. New York: Little, Brown and Company, 2011.

Hever, Julieanna. *The Complete Idiot's Guide to Plant-Based Nutrition*. Indianapolis: Alpha Books, 2011.

Kessler, David A. *The End of Overeating: Controlling the Insatiable American Appetite*. Emmaus, PA: Rodale, 2010.

Lisle, Doug J., and Alan Goldhamer. *The Pleasure Trap: Mastering the Hidden Force That Undermines Health and Happiness*. Summertown, TN: Healthy Living, 2003.

Robbins, John. *Healthy at 100: The Scientifically Proven Secrets of the World's Healthiest and Longest-Lived Peoples*. New York: Ballantine Books, 2007.

———. *The Food Revolution*. San Francisco: Conari Press, 2011.

Stepaniak, Jo. *The Vegan Sourcebook*. Lincolnwood, IL: Lowell House, 2000.

Index

C

H

I-J

X-Y-Z